SpringerBriefs in Applied Sciences and Technology

Forensic and Medical Bioinformatics

Series Editors

Amit Kumar, BioAxis DNA Research Centre Private Ltd, Hyderabad, Telangana, India

Allam Appa Rao, Hyderabad, India

More information about this subseries at http://www.springer.com/series/11910

Nguyen Thi Dieu Linh · Zhongyu (Joan) Lu

Data Science and Medical Informatics in Healthcare Technologies

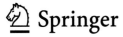

Nguyen Thi Dieu Linh
Hanoi University of Industry
Hanoi, Vietnam

Zhongyu (Joan) Lu
University of Huddersfield
Huddersfield, UK

ISSN 2191-530X   ISSN 2191-5318 (electronic)
SpringerBriefs in Applied Sciences and Technology
ISSN 2196-8845   ISSN 2196-8853 (electronic)
SpringerBriefs in Forensic and Medical Bioinformatics
ISBN 978-981-16-3031-6   ISBN 978-981-16-3029-3 (eBook)
https://doi.org/10.1007/978-981-16-3029-3

This Springer imprint is published by the registered company Springer Nature Singapore Pte Ltd.
The registered company address is: 152 Beach Road, #21-01/04 Gateway East, Singapore 189721, Singapore

Contents

Chapter 1
A Value of Data Science in the Medical Informatics: An Overview

Abstract The use of data science and predictive modelling for real-time clinical decision making is increasingly recognized. The initial step in the path towards the adoption of real-time prediction and forecast is the creation and evaluation of predictive models for clinical practice. Training in medical informatics is not only necessary for medical students but also for all medical personnel at all technical levels of education. A critical move required for the learning and application of clinical medicine is to incorporate medical informatics into the broad scope of medical informatics. Current major fields of research can be categorized according to the organization, implementation, assessment, representation, and interpretation of medical information. We should expect many changes in medical informatics, because of many of the driving forces behind advancement in information management methods and their innovations, developments in medicine and health care, and the constantly evolving needs, requirements and aspirations of human societies. Data science and predictive analytics offer distinct methodologies for tapping vast data sets of medical knowledge from intelligence. These approaches have many possibilities, such as identifying patterns, forecasting outcomes, and optimizing algorithms better. But medical data collection and management often faces few problems, such as data size, data consistency, durability and data completeness. This research offers an extensive overview of medical data processing, predictive analytics and data science in order to contribute to the area of medical informatics and data science. It offers explanations of basic principles using data science in the evolving field of medical informatics. Also the research includes review of benefits, applications and future of data science in healthcare.

Keywords Data science · Medical informatics · Predictive modelling · Healthcare

1.1 Introduction

Statistics research refers to the creation and implementation of instruments for developing, evaluating and interpreting observational medical studies. Innovative use of statistical inference theory, a clear understanding of clinical and epidemiological research problems, and an understanding of the importance of statistical software depend on the development of new statistical methods for medical applications [1]. Strong regulatory and ethical controls, minimum educational credentials, well-established methodologies, compulsory professional accreditation and evidence-based independent review are subject to data science in healthcare. Digital Health, on the other hand, has limited substantive regulation or ethical basis, no defined educational criteria, poor methodologies, a disputed evidence base and negligible peer scrutiny. Yet the vision of 'Big Data' is to base its research on the data that digital health systems create routinely [2]. Industrial companies are dealing with vast volumes of data that Machine Learning requires to understand. Organizations are able to work more effectively and gain advantage over their rivals by gaining information from these results. With Machine Learning algorithms in many fields, groundbreaking predictive models have been implemented successfully. Medical or Health Informatics is a scientific area that deals with the storage, retrieval, and efficient use of medical data, information, and problem-solving and decision-making knowledge. Over the years, health technology has grown tremendously, such as advances in the processing of information, therapies, communication and research [3].

1.2 Predictive Analytics

A new Intel-commissioned report from the International Institute for Analytics found that it is used by the top performers in healthcare analytics to enhance patient participation, population health, and quality of care and business operations, fields that closely map to the Quadruple Aims [4]. However, knowing where to start can be tricky for those not already proficient in analytics. Advanced computational approaches such as machine learning and Artificial Intelligence (AI) offer ground-breaking insights and great breakthrough potential, but they can also be complicated and overwhelming. The best thing is that if you are already on the road to advanced analytics if you are doing some sort of Business Intelligence (BI) today. It is simply a matter of evolution and steady progress from there.

Predictive analytics is the practice of learning from past data in order to formulate predictions about the future. Predictive analytics would allow the right choices to be made for health care, enabling care to be customized to each person. On a bigger scope, physicians have been bringing it into practice. What has improved is our way to evaluate, compile, and make sense of previously complicated or non-existent behavioural, psychosocial, and biometric data. Combining these new datasets with the latest epidemiology and clinical medicine sciences enables us to speed up progress in understanding the interactions between environmental factors and human biology, eventually leading to better clinical pathway reengineering and genuinely personalized treatment. The branch of advanced analytics showing in Fig. 1.1 that is used to make predictions about uncertain future events of big data using data mining, machine learning is predictive analytics [5].

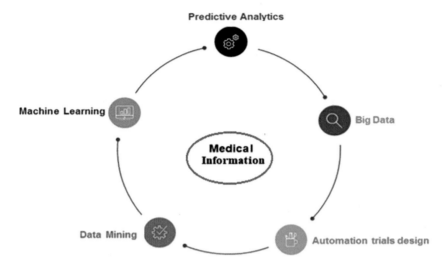

Fig. 1.1 Roles of data science, predictive analysis, ML, and AI in medical information

Predictive analytics employs a variety of applied analytics methods such as data analysis, statistics, modelling, machine learning, and artificial intelligence to interpret existing data and make forecasts about the future. Data learning algorithms and multiple regressions are used to perform predictive analytics sometimes called perspective modelling. The predictor is the main object in predictive analytics, and it is characterized as a variable that is used to measure potential behaviour. With the aid of predictors, potential probabilities are forecasted with incredibly precise outcomes [3].

1.2.1 Analytics-as-a-Service

In the business world, analytics-as-a-service is a relatively newer term compared to data and information-as-a-service. Figure 1.2 shows model management sophistication, service-based analytical model creation and the standardization of the interfaces between models are among the specific challenges that have made analytics-as-a-service a late-emerging effort in information technology [6].

Descriptive analytics. Descriptive analytics often referred to as market reporting, uses the data to address the question of "what happened and/or what is going on?" Easy standard/periodic company reporting, ad-hoc/on-demand reporting and dynamic/interactive reporting are included. Identifying market opportunities and challenges is the key consequence of descriptive analytics.

Predictive analytics. In order to discover explanatory and predictive patterns (trends, correlations, affinities, etc.) reflecting the underlying relationships between data

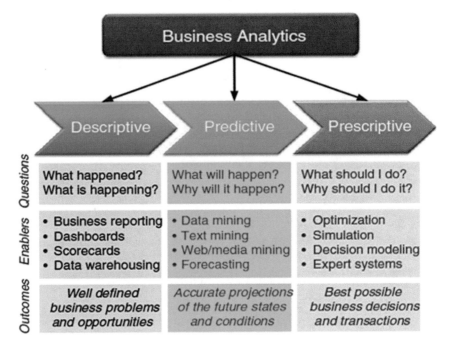

Fig. 1.2 A taxonomy of business analytics [8]

inputs and outputs, predictive analytics uses data and mathematical techniques. In essence, it addresses the problem of "what is going to happen and/or why is it going to happen?" Predictive analytics enablers include data mining, text mining, Web/media mining and forecasting of statistical time series [7].

Prescriptive analytics. In order to evaluate a set of high-value alternative courses of action or decisions, prescriptive analytics uses data and mathematical algorithms given a complex set of goals, criteria and constraints with the objective of optimizing business performance [8].

1.2.2 Predictive Analytics in Healthcare

Prescriptive modelling in healthcare uses past evidence to make potential forecasts, customizing treatment for each individual. The past medical background, demographic details and actions of a person can be used to forecast the future in accordance with the skills and experience of healthcare professionals. Computer tools do not describe healthcare predictive analytics, reflecting the current technology wave to advance the industry. The merely difference is that quite a few years ago, physician's minds were predicting the facts based on their experience and expertise. Today, software tools are used to analyzing the data to perform the predictions [7].

1.2.3   Predictive Analytics and Healthcare

At lightning speed, the healthcare industry is changing. Predictive analytics is the primary goal, generating immense opportunities to optimize patient outcomes and minimize costs. To model future outcomes, predictive analytics uses past data. It would probably help to classify patients at the greatest risk of adverse health outcomes. Via remote patient control, it can also aid in providing personalized treatment. In order to reduce hospitalization and re-admissions, physicians should target these care receivers with personalized health plans. Specialists may harness innovation to draw valuable conclusions for disease study, such as big data analytics, machine learning algorithms, and natural language processing. In turn, this will allow patients to take part in their own care. At the very least, before they escalate, this type of analytics will help clinicians predict issues before creating and mitigating health problems. It is proving to be a crucial competitive advantage for companies today when you combine predictive analytics and big data.

1.2.4   Machine Learning's Role in Predictions

Enterprises are encouraged to see greater meaning in the massive amounts of data they collect and save every day. Machine learning architectures, tools, and applications are introduced to attain optimal predictive accuracy and value for organization's sets of data, as well as lead to the effectiveness of different strategies. Machine learning methods are designed to discover the potential to improve decisions based on the predictive nature of large-scale data sets. It shows that predictive tasks, like determining which behaviours appear to drive desired outcomes, are successful in managing them [3].

1.3   The Role of Data Science in Healthcare

Data science describes a class of techniques designed to allow computers, as humans do, to feel, reason, act, and adapt. Data science is made up of many underlying technologies. Think of these as several instruments that can be used to solve different forms of data issues. As data science becomes more complex, some of these technologies would probably be needed as part of an end-to-end solution [4]. Healthcare services have a plethora of essential yet vulnerable data. A diverse collection of data such as basic demographics, identified disorders, and a wealth of clinical knowledge such as findings from laboratory tests are contained in medical records. For patients with chronic conditions, due to the frequency of visits to a healthcare provider, a long and comprehensive history of data on a variety of health metrics may be available. Patient records information may also be mixed with outside data as well [9].

For instance, to calculate the number of surgeons who work near a patient or other specific information about the type of area in which patients live, a patient's address may be combined with other publicly accessible information.

Models can be developed and trained to predict several outcomes of interest with this rich data about a patient as well as their environment. Models that predict disease progression, which can be used for disease management and planning, are one significant field of interest. For instance, a chronic kidney disease progression model at Fresenius medical which can forecast the course of a patient's condition to help clinicians determine whether and when to continue with their medical care to the next level. In order to reduce the likelihood of unfavourable effects, predictive models may also alert clinicians about patients who may need treatments. We use models, for example, to predict which patients are at risk of hospitalization or lack of dialysis care. These predictions are provided to clinicians, along with the main factors influencing the prediction, who may determine whether certain treatments will help reduce the risk of the patient [10].

Medical informatics is a type of data science that incorporates biotechnology and clinical facets, as well as medical information and technologies in social, behavioral, governance, policy, and other areas. While it has been used for decades in bioinformatics, health data science is a recent name that emerged with the emergence of large medical information. In fact, in the earlier years of biomedical informatics, medical data science was perhaps the most important topic. Because of recent advances in computer learning, data analytics, and computation resources. Medical data science is recently experiencing a revival, eventually able to solve some of the toughest real-world issues. In general, the field of biomedical informatics is an interdisciplinary field involving the following [11]:

Clinical science and practice: Population health, medicine, dentistry, nursing, pharmacy, Public and community health.

Engineering in computer science: Databases, scripting algorithms, neural networks, artificial intelligence, semantic computing, computer learning (including deep learning), cloud computing, text and natural language processing,, surveillance, distributed computing visualization, sensors, Internet of Things (IoT), mobile devices, social networks, and so on are all examples of technology.

Cognitive science: Cognitive psychology, linguistics, behavioural science, and artificial intelligence are only a few examples.

Biostatistics: Biostatistics is a branch of statistics whose primary aim is to advance statistical analysis and its application to human health and disease issues.

Social and behavioural sciences: The social and behavioural sciences observe and inspect healthcare data to find out the tendency in health-related behaviours, together with the occurrence of unhealthy behaviours.

Management science: Healthcare Data Management facilitates to combine and analyze Healthcare data to make patient care more proficient, and extract insights that can improve medical outcomes, while protecting the security and privacy of the data.

1.3.1 Benefits of Data Science in Healthcare

Data Science aims to advance procedures and services for health care. It helps to maximize diagnostic and treatment efficiency and improve the workflow of healthcare systems. The healthcare system's ultimate priorities are as follows [12]:

- To ease the health-care system workflow.
- To minimize the risk of failure of care.
- To have adequate counselling on time.
- To prevent needless emergencies due to the inaccessibility of doctors.
- To decrease patients' waiting time.

1.3.2 The Role of a Data Scientist in Healthcare

The task of a data scientist is to incorporate all data science techniques to integrate them into healthcare software. To make predictive models, the data scientist extracts valuable insights from the data. Overall, a DATA SCIENTIST's healthcare commitments are as follows [13]:

- Gathering patient data.
- Analysis of hospitals' needs.
- Structuring and arranging the details for use.
- Doing data analytics using different instruments.
- Implementing data algorithms for extracting insights.
- Construction with the development team of predictive models.

1.3.3 Challenges of Data Science in Healthcare

One challenge is that, in terms of embracing the new technologies and analytics tools, the healthcare industry is well behind other industries. This poses some difficulties, and data scientists should be mindful that, in many healthcare organizations, the data technology and development landscape will not be at the cutting edge of the industry. It also implies, however, that there are many opportunities for improvement, and even small, simple models can produce substantial improvements over existing methods.

The confidential nature of medical knowledge poses another problem in the healthcare field. It can also be difficult to gain access to data that the organization has because of concerns about data privacy. For this reason, data scientists seeking a job in a healthcare organization should be aware of whether a protocol for data professionals to gain access to data is already in place. If there isn't, be mindful that it could be a big undertaking in itself to simply get access to the data. Finally, the end-use of any predictive model is necessary to bear in mind. In certain ways, false-negatives and false-positives have somewhat different costs. A false negative can be harmful to the wellbeing of a patient, while too many false positives may lead to many expensive and needless procedures (also to the detriment of the health of patients for such treatments as well as the overall economy). For end-users, knowledge about the correct use of predictive models and their drawbacks is important. Finally, it is necessary to make sure the performance of a predictive model is actionable. It is only useful to predict that a patient is at high risk if the model outputs are interpretable enough to understand what factors put the patient at risk. In addition, if the model is used to design treatments, it is important to illustrate the variables that can be altered in any way-telling a clinician that a patient is at risk because of their age is not helpful if the point of the forecast is to minimize risk through intervention [11].

1.3.4 Applications of Data Science in Healthcare

Drug Research. As the world's population is rising, every now and then there are many problems in a human body arising. This may be due to the lack of adequate food, anxiety, pollution, physical diseases, etc. Seeking drugs or vaccines for diseases in a short span of time has now become a problem for medical research institutes. Since researchers have to consider the characteristics of the causative agent to find a formula for a drug, it may take millions of test cases to do this. Then, the researchers have to conduct more experiments on the formula after discovering a formula. It took 10–12 years to go through the data from the millions of test cases listed above, in earlier days. But, now, it has become a much easier challenge with the aid of different data science applications in healthcare. Data may be analyzed within months or can be in weeks from millions of test cases. It helps to assess the drug's efficiency by analyzing data. The vaccine or medication successfully tested can therefore be released in less than a year. With the assistance of data science and machine learning, this is all possible. All have revolutionised the medicinal drug industry's research and development industries. Next, we can see data science's use in genomics [14].

Virtual Assistance. A perfect example of the use of data science is the applications that are developed using virtual assistance. Data scientists have developed robust systems that provide patients with individualized experience. The medical apps that use data science aid a patient by evaluating the symptoms to classify the illness. The patient just needs to have his/her symptoms and the application will predict the patient's illness and condition. Precautions, medication, and the care needed according to the patient's condition [14] will be suggested. In addition, the program analyzes the patient's data and generates a checklist of the treatment processes to be followed. Then, the patient is periodically informed about taking drugs. This helps to eliminate a neglect incident that may make the condition worse.

Tracking and Preventing Diseases. Data Science plays a key role in tracking the health of patients and notifying them of the appropriate measures to be taken to prevent the outbreak of possible diseases. Data scientists use powerful predictive analytical methods at an early stage to diagnose chronic diseases. There are instances of negligibility in certain serious cases; diseases are not caught at an early stage [8]. This is particularly detrimental to not only the welfare of the patient, but also to the economic costs. The price of treating it also rises as the disease progresses. Therefore, in maximizing economic spending on healthcare, data science plays a huge role. We may conclude that data science is one of the wonderful inventions of human beings by looking at all these applications of data science in healthcare. So, we conclude that in healthcare, data science has many applications. Data science has been heavily used by the medicine and healthcare industry to change patients' lives and predict diseases at an early level. In addition, with developments in medical image processing, it is possible for physicians to classify microscopic tumours that would otherwise be difficult to locate. Data science has, thus, revolutionised healthcare and the medical industry in large ways.

Data Management and Data Governance. The opportunity is immense for improved data management. Moving for greater use of open standards and better top-level exchange of data offers actionable insights into the functioning of the health service. Machine learning would encourage physicians to be more compassionate and to provide better treatment. Data management is all about making data readily available to individuals in the healthcare sector who work. As the essence of the health industry is risk-entailing, to determine the current situation and future effects, data crunching needs to be ultra-careful. In addition, healthcare data analytics should remain up-to-date, complete, and profound. The method is supported by data science for healthcare:

- All Electronic Health Records (EHR) can be compiled into one dataset, stored in the information distribution centre and used effortlessly for the planning and testing of the resulting model.
- All information can be digitized, gathered, and exchanged over different data sets and systematized, reducing unnecessary office work.
- Extra sources and further review can assist in recognizing and handling the clinical knowledge gap.
- Cloud-based healthcare software provides options for usability and accelerates the data handling process. It means saving time when deciding on therapy or obtaining results from the laboratory.

Although data governance is recognized as an imperative for healthcare, there are opportunities for healthcare organizations to hasten data governance prioritization as a business imperative. The concept includes laws, procedures, processes, tasks, and responsibilities for data lifecycle management. Data governance offers guidelines in its essence to ensure that information is reliable, consistent, complete, accessible, and safe. It is also a key enabler to improve data value and confidence and to achieve efficiencies and cost savings. In patient involvement, coordination of care, and community health, data governance plays a key role. The data would be published inconsistently by numerous healthcare data science firms without it. In exchange, this would contribute to the impression of low data quality. Healthcare data science apps therefore ensure a more reliable approach to security and a deeper study of the system [14].

Workflow Optimization and Process Improvements. It's a little-known fact that with human 'gut instinct' many major decisions are made, as there are few big data analytics in healthcare. Medical data science enables a customized approach to healthcare to be created and allows healthcare organizations more effectively manage time and workload [15]. This is how the workflow is enhanced by data science:

- Knowledge bases and distributed computing functions will dramatically shorten the time needed for the operation and improve the accuracy of the test results.
- Less time and reliable test results contribute to the improvement of work process performance.
- Medical workers are ultimately granted the ability to perform further duties within a short amount of time.
- Better performance leads to higher recovery rates, quicker incident response, and, above all, fewer fatal outcomes due to sepsis and multiple components that require a rapid response.
- Recipients of health care get digital contact that is patient-cantered.

Furthermore, data science instruments promote a superior system for the general advancement of the human services framework. Each test, evaluation, guess, and treatment involves another case for machine learning algorithms, reinforcing the logical limits of the worldwide social insurance system.

Medical Image Analysis. For clinical diagnosis and medical intervention, medical imaging refers to the method of producing a visual image of the body. It provides a non-invasive way for doctors before a surgery to look inside the human body, or model organs. With the exponential growth of healthcare and artificial intelligence, data science technologies in healthcare will play a key role in developing new treatment and care opportunities. Tomography or longitudinal tomography is among the different forms of medical imaging. X-ray, Computer Tomography (CT), Positron Emission Tomography (PET), and Magnetic Resonance Imaging (MRI) are its principal techniques. Anyway, how is the science of data changing healthcare in that area? Well, accurate images with subsequent meticulous analysis are needed for medical imaging. Image processing refines image analysis by developing such features as:

- Modality difference
- Image size
- Resolution

By providing computational capabilities that process images at scale with greater speed and precision, supervised and unsupervised learning enables medical imaging.

The data sets are the cornerstones of the examination, and their large libraries. The data entry is compared to the available datasets, and the gathered bits of information provide a superior understanding of the diagnosis of the patients.

Genetics/Genomics—Treatment personalization. Whether it's different ways of genomic profiling sequencing or something else, this gives a fresh look at the genomics environment as new innovations come along. With enormous quantities of data today, genetic knowledge is now generated faster than it can be organized or implemented. Part of this is because the strategies for structuring information lag significantly behind improving the capacity to collect information. Data science for healthcare is a positive idea, so you have to be able to make sense of it. In the genomics sector, the challenges include the following:

- Studying human genetic variation and its effect on patients
- Identifying genetic risk factors for drug response.

Predictive analytics. Predictive analytics is basically a technology that learns from experience to predict the potential behaviour of a patient. By drawing accurate conclusions about current and future events, it helps tie health care data science to meaningful action. In addition to use models used in data science medicine, predictive analytics enables healthcare to use predictive models. This, in turn, allows possible threats and opportunities to be detected before they arise. Here, however, are some challenges to the use of predictive analytics. These include points that are as follows:

- Lack of smooth sharing of healthcare information between systems and personnel
- Shortage of trained staff to fill the holes in expertise
- To remove these obstacles and encourage the use of predictive analysis, the following types of databases are required
- Medical history
- Patients' ongoing condition stats
- Lists of prescription
- Genetic analysis and other applications.

Combined, the process will skyrocket through data retrieval and deep learning:

- Techniques of data mining derive useful data from large batches of data.
- Illustrative, exploratory and comparative calculations will incorporate different points of view into one and determine the best choice for patients.

In general, analytics of this kind can:

- Provide fast and precise insights to make use of risk scores
- Enhance organizational performance
- Prediction of outbreak
- Monitor the deterioration of patients
- Reducing the cost of waste elimination and fraud
- Predicting the cost of insurance products through the application of data science in health insurance.

Therefore, patients have the potential advantage of improved performance due to predictive analytics [16]. At the same time, it will also allow the healthcare industry to establish forecasting models that do not involve a lot of cases.

1.3.5 Future of Data Science in Healthcare Domain

Basically, in the healthcare sector, there are four factors contributing to rapid improvement:

- Technical changes
- Digitalisation
- Need for dropping treatment duration and costs
- Need for managing huge population.

At present time, to minimize the cost and length of treatment necessity to control large populations is an important requirement. Data Science has already begun to resolve all of these in order to have the desired impact. There is no question that its implementation in the future will prove to be more invaluable, since Data Science is already doing wonders for society. The healthcare sector will push it to more heights. Doctors are given enough assistance and patients are given a more personalized experience and services that are ideal. In healthcare, the future holds a lot of promise for data science. Wearable devices that track all sorts of behaviour and biometric information are becoming more advanced and more prevalent. Streaming data from either wearable or therapeutic devices (such as dialysis machines) could potentially be used to provide patients or clinicians with real-time warnings about health incidents outside the hospital [2].

Today, a big problem facing medical professionals is that data from patients continues to remain in silos. There is little integration among medical providers through electronic medical record systems is required, which can contribute to fragmented treatment in a better way. This may result in clinicians receiving obsolete or incomplete patient records, or duplication of therapies. These schemes could be integrated through a major data engineering initiative. This would significantly expand the ability of data scientists and data engineers, who could then offer analytics services and provide a degree of continuity across care facilities, taking into account the full history of patients. Such an automated record may be used by data staff to alert physicians to duplicate procedures or unsafe combinations of prescription drugs. Within the healthcare sector, data scientists have a lot to give. In a place where people's wellbeing can be strengthened, developments in machine learning and data science can and should be embraced. In this field, the prospects for data scientists are almost infinite, and the potential for good is immense. In the healthcare field, data analytics and predictive modelling have immense potential for the future showing in Fig. 1.3. With the aid of wearable equipment that can monitor an individual's results, it is promising. These devices are used to monitor biometric information and to make biometric data more advanced and extremely popular.

Medical & patient data
Electronic Health Records (EHR) health sensors, social media, and genomics create rich new data sources for analytics

Big data analytics
Cheap computing power and sophisticated analytics drive insights into patient behavior, treatment costs and R&D

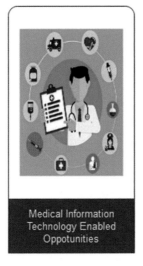

Moblie/mHealth
Pervasive mobile and smart phone adoption creates new engagement models within daily routines

Health care professionals digital workflow
Increasing integration of EHRs and telehealth drives new digitally-enabled coordinated workforce models of care

Influence patients behaviors beyond the pill' and sustain engagement outside the traditional care setting

Medical Information Technology Enabled Oppotunities

Discover and deliver targeted and personalised therapies with real-world evidence of impact

Fig. 1.3 How data analysis and predictive model is used in health care

The data is streamed in real-time with the aid of certain care devices or wearable devices that can give a health status warning to a doctor outside the premises of a hospital or clinic [17]. The biggest challenge faced by medical suppliers is that the data continues to exist in the storage tower. For these major medical electronic records that result in the fragmented treatment of data, the incorporation is not commonly used. The consequence of this procedure is that a doctor or clinician receives incomplete or obsolete patient records.

They might also be eligible to undergo care. However, this scheme can be integrated such that, with the aid of data engineering, data can be reliable and appropriate. This single tweaking shifts the landscape of this industry and will have a major effect on the workload. The imminent involvement of computer engineers and data scientists will increase. They can then provide more precise analytical services that take into account the more consistent outcome of a patient's entire health condition. The problem of data replication, prescribing of any unsafe medications, or procedures will be eliminated by this method [18, 19].

- We also read how much promise data science and predictive model can have in the area of healthcare.
- It can add to the industry's expertise with small tricks and tips, as described above. We have, however, summarized a few big ways that will continue to improve the value of healthcare data science and predictive modelling.
- Now, by sending a warning to the respective clinic or hospital, it is possible to put wearable devices in use that can track, monitor and even avoid any heart-related condition.

- With the aid of monitoring history and correctly predicting the outcomes with efficiency, it is a perfect way to enhance a patient's diagnosis.
- It is now better to transform patient care into precision medicine that can track and monitor the history of symptoms and treatment before delivering accurate outcomes.
- With the aid of pharmaceutical science, this scheme is moving towards the cure of chronic diseases.
- It will help to optimize clinical efficiency that will not have to endure all the data and with the help of diagnosis, the machine will provide insight into the problem.

1.4 Conclusion

Data science has been transformed in recent years from academic curiosity to a broad industry in healthcare informatics and medical data processing. The healthcare data analytics and informatics helps advanced treatment strategies and enhance medical outcomes. For today's healthcare industry, an increased emphasis on best practices and technology solutions that capture, process and interpret data is crucial and creating new opportunities for organizations with data analytics and health informatics expertise. The need to develop and apply new methods for the efficient integration, review and interpretation of complex healthcare data in order to establish testable hypotheses and develop detailed models for diagnosing and predicting different types of diseases. In this study benefits, challenges and applications of data science in healthcare is considered. Also role of data science and predictive analysis in medical informatics have been discussed. In order to achieve best outcomes of medical informatics using data science there is a need to develop more optimized and accurate predictive analytics methods.

References

1. P. Nieminen, Applications of medical informatics and data analysis methods. MDPI, Applied Science **10**, 7359 (2020)
2. P.J. Scott, R. Dunscombe, D. Evans, J.C. Wyatt, M. Mukherjee, Learning health systems need to bridge the 'two cultures' of clinical informatics and data science. J. Innov. Health Inform. **25**(2) (2018)
3. B. Nithya, V. Ilango, Predictive analytics in health care using machine learning tools and techniques, in *International Conference on Intelligent Computing and Control Systems ICICCS 2017*
4. A. Bartley, Predictive analytics in healthcare, White paper on Healthcare Predictive Analytics © Intel Corporation
5. A. Kankanhalli, J. Hahn, S. Tan, G. Gao, Big data and analytics in healthcare: introduction to the special section. Inf. Syst. Front. **18**(2), 233–235 (2016)
6. D.W. Bates, S. Saria, L. Ohno-Machado, A. Shah, G. Escobar, Big data in health care: using analytics to identify and manage high-risk and high-cost patients. Health Aff. **33**(7), 1123–1131 (2014)

7. G. Palem, The Practice of Predictive Analytics in Healthcare (2013). https://www.researchg ate.net/publication/236336250
8. D. Delen, H. Demirkan, Data, information and analytics as services, © 2012 Elsevier, May 2012
9. E. Bruballa, A. Wong, F. Epelde, D. Rexachs, E. Luque, A model to predict length of stay in a hospital emergency department and enable planning for non-critical patients admission. Int. J. Integr. Care **16**(6), 1–2 (2016)
10. M. Barad, T. Hadas, R.A. Yarom, H. Weisman, Emergency department crowding, in *19th IEEE International Conference on Emerging Technologies and Factory Automation, ETFA* (2014)
11. I.D. Dinov, Methodological challenges and analytic opportunities for modelling and interpreting Big Healthcare Data. Gigascience **5**(1), 12 (2016)
12. H. Asri, H. Mousannif, H. Al Moatassime, T. Noel, Big data in healthcare: challenges and opportunities, in *Proceedings of 2015 International Conference on Cloud Computer Technology Application CloudTech* (2015)
13. W. Raghupathi, V. Raghupathi, Big data analytics in healthcare: promise and potential. Heal. Inf. Sci. Syst. **2**(1), 3 (2014)
14. M. Ojha, K. Mathur, Proposed application of big data analytics in healthcare at Maharaja Yeshwantrao Hospital, in *3rd MEC International Conference on Big Data and Smart City (ICBDSC)* (2016), pp. 1–7
15. R. Chauhan, R. Jangade, A robust model for big healthcare data analytics, in *6th International Conference—Cloud System and Big Data Engineering (Confluence)* (2016), pp. 221–225
16. J.D. Sonis, E.L. Aaronson, R.Y. Lee, L.L. Philpotts, B.A. White, Emergency department patient experience. J. Patient Exp. **5**(2), 101–106 (2018)
17. Y. Sun, K.L. Teow, B.H. Heng, C.K. Ooi, S.Y. Tay, Real-time prediction of waiting time in the emergency department, using quantile regression. Ann. Emerg. Med. **60**(3), 299–308 (2012)
18. R. Ding, M.L. McCarthy, J. Lee, J.S. Desmond, S.L. Zeger, D. Aronsky, Predicting emergency department length of stay using quantile regression. Int. Conf. Manage. Serv. Sci. **45**(2), 1–4 (2009)
19. A.T. Janke, D.L. Overbeek, K.E. Kocher, P.D. Levy, Exploring the potential of predictive analytics and big data in emergency care. Ann. Emerg. Med. **67**(2), 227–236 (2016)

Chapter 2
Data Science in Medical Informatics: Challenges and Opportunities

Abstract The healthcare system is undergoing a significant transition, necessitated by the triple goal of improving efficiency, lower costs and improving outcomes. Healthcare analytics may be implemented at different levels, including monitoring and avoiding medical errors, data integration, predictive analysis and personalized modelling. Although substantial advancement and progress has been made from the perspective of data science and study, challenges and opportunities remain. Current major fields of study can be categorized according to the organisation, implementation and assessment of health information systems, the representation of medical information and the analysis and interpretation of underlying signals and data. We can anticipate many changes in future medical informatics science, considering the fluid existence of many of the driving forces behind innovation in information processing methods and their technology, advancement in medicine and health care, and the rapidly evolving needs, requirements and desires of human societies. This chapter consists of opportunities and challenges of data science in healthcare information analysis. Also data analytics stages, future and its technologies are briefly discussed.

Keywords Data science · Predictive analysis · Medical informative · Healthcare analysis

2.1 Introduction

As with advances in time and technology, in order to improve the efficiency, effectiveness and effectiveness of medical treatment, a structural improvement in health systems is required. The strategic mission of Value-based Health Care is to ensure that everyone can make use of the health services required for their healthy health and well-being. Focus on value-based treatment leads to an expanded emphasis on patient care. Doctors, physicians and health providers must collaborate together to personalize care that is efficient, effective in quality and billing, and measure it on the basis of patient satisfaction by concentrating on patient experiences in technologies and healthcare processes. In order to improve the reliability and safety of patient care [1], the introduction of electronic health records and the comprehensive processing

© The Author(s), under exclusive license to Springer Nature Singapore Pte Ltd. 2021 17
N. Thi Dieu Linh and Z. (Joan). Lu, *Data Science and Medical Informatics in Healthcare Technologies*, SpringerBriefs in Forensic and Medical Bioinformatics,
https://doi.org/10.1007/978-981-16-3029-3_2

of data by health care providers have been planned. Statistics research relates to the creation and application of instruments for the design, study and evaluation of observational medical studies. The imaginative use of statistical inference theory, a strong understanding of the problems of clinical and epidemiological study and an understanding of the importance of statistical software depend on the development of new statistical approaches for medical applications [2].

In nearly every region of the economy, data analytics has become increasingly relevant. A complex variety of private and public data collection programs with various data sources are involved in health care. As health care services moved to Electronic Health Records (EHRs), multimedia laboratory images, and high-resolution radiology videos and photos, the number of data grew exponentially in the previous century. Data petabytes are stored in health care providers' libraries, and trillions of data points are streamed from monitors such as fitness trackers and various other continuous tracking systems. Healthcare digitization results in the development of vast new data sets. The Electronic Medical Record (EMR) is one of the most important instances of this. More than 85% of United States's healthcare organizations have now accepted an EMR system [3].

Other common data sets are insurance claims data, radiology pictures and lab outcomes. Knowledge on genomics is expected to expand dramatically in the future as precision medicine is gradually incorporated into routine clinical practice workflows. Via the usage of wearable health and wellness trackers and mobile apps, the healthcare industry produces a large amount of health data outside of the healthcare systems. Every day, the expansion of health-related Internet of Things (IoT) applications, as well as smartphone and other health-monitoring technology, provides a tremendous quantity of data. Healthcare companies have a huge opportunity to merge all disparate data sets and processes into new technologies. In addition to patient data, it is essential to remember population health trends using external information such as social media or widely accessible government information. However, 94% of hospitals do not actually gather sufficient information to perform a productive population health analysis [4]. In the following section, challenges and opportunities faced by healthcare data analytics are discussed.

2.1.1   Challenges

Analytics. In data collection and management, there are several problems resulting from incomplete, heterogeneous, inaccurate, or inconsistent data. For efficient data analytics, the principle of core attribute values focused on high utility value and cost effectiveness is crucial. The challenges in dealing with such a huge number of possible predictors, as well as the rarity of many of the cases of concern, must be addressed. The difficulties of dealing with a large number of possible predictors, as well as the rarity of each of the events of concern, must be addressed by certain analytics [5]. As organisations collaborate and exchange information to enable an integrated EMR, privacy becomes critical. For the purposes of statistical modelling and population studies, privacy must be maintained when sharing information and maintaining much of the usefulness of aggregated data while adhering to privacy limitations. When data from various sources is combined, the privacy-utility tradeoffs become much more important to consider, potentially leading to unintended effects or leaks.

Adoption of Technology. The key roadblocks to predictive modelling's acceptance and deployment in healthcare can be broken down into two stages: adoption and product use. The first is due to a lack of awareness of its utility as well as an inability to stick to strategic goals. Health professionals are overworked, and there has been no incentive to look at how analytics can help them be more efficient and successful. Data access and sharing capabilities are often limited by privacy and sensitivity concerns associated with patient information. In challenging clinical workflows, processes, and environments, the second set of problems is correlated with real device use. When dealing with electronic medical records on a regular basis, clinicians face a number of challenges. Some barriers to usability include a lack of support for data synchronization, fragmentation of data, too many choices for each area, a lack of overview visual analytics, exchange of information in a privacy-safe manner, and so on. While EMRs provide help for organized data entry, due to the lack of system accessibility and time, clinicians frequently revert to unstructured notes. This causes problems with natural language decoding as well as data errors. More importantly, the complexity of primary EMR usage leads to a lack of faith in their efficacy, resulting in a lack of interest in their secondary and potentially more effective use, namely clinical predictive analysis.

Lack of Involvement of Data Scientists. Traditionally, clinicians relied heavily on biostatisticians for analysis and understanding. Technology from large-scale data analytical tools in other industries can be implemented as data processing capabilities evolve and large volumes of data are collected. It is also extremely important to exploit the expertise of data scientists when designing analytical solutions. Therefore, leveraging the expertise of data scientists when designing analytical solutions is increasingly necessary. Acceptance and integration of these skills has been sluggish in the health system as a whole, with the potential exception of payers, but there is an increasing awareness of the need [6].

2.1.2 Opportunities

Compared to other industries, such as finance and banking, the problems listed above, along with other legal and regulatory constraints, make healthcare a late-accepter of technology. While many technical concerns are of concern, the key possibilities include [7]:

Research Opportunities. Research opportunities: It will be important to integrate domain expertise and real world evidence to tackle data quality problems to further enhance the efficacy of predictive modelling follow-up efforts. It would be important to pick function techniques, because most healthcare data is of very large dimensions. In the integration of proof from various sources, smart ensemble approaches can play a crucial role. Finally, for effective cooperation and for the incorporation of data from various sources, knowledge-preserving data sharing and privacy-aware techniques are important. The harmonization of data elements through data collection schemes is one of the most significant challenges. It may provide new opportunities for epidemiological research to achieve consensus about what is assessed. What is assessed will determine what concerns get clinical attention in the clinical practice arena.

Addressing the Needs of Practitioners Inside Their Workflow. The emphasis of approaches should be on making practices smarter and simpler to deal with for doctors. A system that illustrates key points in a document format and responds to clinicians' questions when reading medical records, for example, would allow doctors to concentrate on patient care rather than data collection and analysis. Usability and efficiency will be the driving forces behind technology acceptance.

Interdisciplinary Design Teams. While there is a strong consensus on the need for doctors and data scientists to work together and cooperate on the creation and production of successful IT solutions, a more coherent and cohesive interdisciplinary team of practitioners, data scientists, biostatisticians, policy makers, legal experts, etc. is required. Otherwise, most healthcare structures would inevitably be designed into a narrow framework that does not provide viable alternatives, leading to dissatisfaction and loss of faith in the success of these systems.

Considerations, prospects, and obstacles of using data analytics to incorporate healthcare informatics are addressed in this section. This topic isn't meant to be exhaustive; rather, it's meant to illustrate particular issues in order to highlight the need for a well-thought-out collection of best practices to drive the rise of data science in healthcare. It will aid in meeting the aims of bettering outcomes, enhancing clinical practice, and lowering health-care costs. However, new problems that have arisen as a result of the advancement of existing technology must be addressed.

2.2 Data Science in Healthcare

Without a question, Machine Learning (ML), data science and Artificial Intelligence (AI) have become hot topics in all fields, including healthcare. Companies are scrambling to stock up on data scientists, big and small, but are data scientists alone enough to create a strong healthcare data science practice? Data scientists are, without a doubt, needed to create models. But you need an entire ecosystem of support functions to grow and maintain the team while you are dealing with healthcare and human data [7]. Big data analytics refers to the massive amounts of data that have been accessible to healthcare providers since the industry's digitization. Actionable insights can be extracted from a comprehensive review of these data sets,

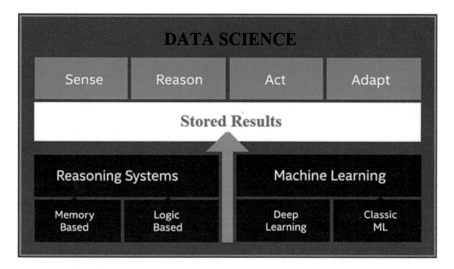

Fig. 2.1 Technologies behind data science

causing better action to be made on healthcare problems. This leads to the production of detailed and holistic experiences of patients, clients, and doctors. Data Science is applied to a variety of technologies, as seen in Fig. 2.1. Data science can also be used efficiently for health informatics by using context technology.

Data-driven decision making opens up new possibilities for healthcare quality enhancement. A few handpicked cases of using data science in healthcare are described below.

Improve Diagnostic Accuracy
A new study has shown that 12 million patients are misdiagnosed annually in the United States and 10% of deaths occur due to medical errors [8]. Healthcare professionals can enhance diagnostic precision and decrease mortality rates by unlocking the supremacy of data analytics. Through making use of sophisticated data analysis technologies and machine learning algorithms to increase diagnosis accuracy, a range of data analytics firms are now offering solutions to providers. Predictive computational methods analyze historical evidence, including case data, health notes, signs, behaviours, illnesses, genome structure, etc., in order to forecast the results accurately.

Make Use of EHR More Effective
Electronic Health Records (EHRs) are a digital archive containing patient information that can be downloaded by authorized patients at any time. Since the most recent data, over than 95% of hospitals and almost 90% of office-based doctors have implemented the EHR method [8]. The availability of digital backups of medical records has become a game-changing shift in the healthcare sector, and perhaps one of the most common applications of big data. EHR use has many advantages,

including lower costs, improved patient efficiency, and streamlined procedures. The McKinsey report 'The Big Data Revolution in US Healthcare-Accelerating Value and Innovation' applies to the health link example, which enables the exchange of information across all medical facilities and promotes the use of EHR.

Analyze Medical Images Efficiently

Another important industry that profits from big data and analytics is medical imaging. Last year, almost 600 million monitoring and assessment were performed in the United States alone [8]. Without disk retrieval facilities, any of this data will be difficult to store manually. Deep learning models are being used to assess differences in X-Ray, medical examinations, tomography, mammography and other medical imaging methods in terms of modality, size and resolution. This enables physicians to improve diagnostic accuracy, recognize various illnesses, and aid in the identification of better care alternatives.

Create Effective Pharmaceutical Drugs in a Shorter Period

Finding a new prescription drug necessitates a variety of treatments and tests, as well as a significant amount of time and money. With the emergence of big data analytics, researchers will automate and speed up this process. Data analytics and deep learning algorithms have a data-driven perspective to research classes at any stage of the process. It will predict the performance level and how the substance would behave in the human body, resulting in more precise drug manufacturing. Furthermore, genetic science necessitates the development of computational drugs to understand how chemical molecules respond to various cell types, gene abnormalities, and other factors. Data science applications are also a spark for a new era of pharmaceutical research.

Reduce Risks in Prescription Medicine

Data science research seeks to reduce the dangers associated with prescription medications as well as to improve diagnosis accuracy. Deep-learning algorithms compare with the available databases as a prescription is offered to the patient and alert the doctor if it deviates from standard care protocols. Health care services benefit from this by optimizing medical quality and avoiding deadly complications associated with faulty drugs.

To Trigger Real-time Alerts

In-house healthcare is costly, as we have recognized, but recording the patient's health statistics is very much required for better care. With the introduction of wearable technology, clinicians can virtually monitor the patient's vital statistics and, where applicable, offer real-time medical assistance. Wearable sensors record and store patient records in a cloud that is open to treatment administrators and suppliers. For example, the system warns the physician who may take urgent measures to save the patient when there is a disturbing change in the blood pressure of the patient.

Improve Patient Engagement

A value-based treatment strategy is practiced by today's healthcare providers, and patient participation plays a major role in it. Raising the role of patients in the recovery plan has since been a top priority for healthcare providers. In order to satisfy the demands of the tech-savvy patient community, they engage primarily in developing methods. To ensure that patients are fully engaged in their treatment, healthcare professionals can easily implement big data analytics. To increase treatment alignment, artificial intelligence natural language processing and machine learning can be used to extract actionable lessons and produce predictive risk scores. It mostly serves people enrolled in chronic disease care services.

Streamline Knowledge Management

Problem-solving and achieving desired healthcare outcomes depend largely on the information bank. In the current healthcare environment, handling both internal expertise and externally gained knowledge efficiently is a challenge for the provider. An effective knowledge management approach is important for delivering the best care possible, achieving organizational excellence, and boosting innovation. It is easier to compile, store and distribute multiple medical facts with the introduction of big data into healthcare. Data science techniques are capable of integrating knowledge from different sources in order to achieve maximum organizational efficiency, and providers can use analytics.

Simplify Internal Staffing Process

Through mathematical analyses, it is easy to calculate how often people are already in the hospital on a regular and even hourly basis. It helps in streamlining the overall workforce management process, resulting in reduced patient wait times and improved service quality. Personnel planners in any healthcare company struggle to estimate the number of workers anticipated at any specified period. If the percentage of jobs is higher than predicted, there will be a labor shortage, and if the number of staff is lower, there will be poor customer service.

Reduce Visits to Doctor

With the help of artificial intelligence, smartphone devices are now in a position to provide the necessary resources for health care. Instead of waiting for a doctor's appointment, patients will explain their conditions, ask questions, and at any time take tips and recommendations from smart chatbots. It provides timely updates of the medications and recovery plans and also helps to schedule a doctor's appointment. For both patients and doctors, AI-based applications are useful. Since it saves doctors time and can deal with more urgent situations, patients receive round-the-clock assistance. It encourages the patient to follow a healthier lifestyle that ultimately leads to enhanced health outcomes.

Find a Cure for Deadly Diseases

One of the many potential applications of health data science is to identify treatments for dangerous diseases such as cancer, Ebola, etc. An immense volume of evidence is available to researchers on care strategies, survival rates, disease symptoms, mortality, etc. They will uncover patterns and therapies that deliver high success rates in the real world by using data analytics technology. Drug researchers can, for example, investigate how certain mutations and cancer proteins combine to find the best combination to save the patient. In order to improve the quality of treatment, hospital facilities are continually looking for new solutions. It has adopted emerging technology in a timely way and aims to develop for a better future. A change in the making is Big Data in healthcare. The way patients, doctors, and healthcare providers view the delivery of care has just begun to shift [7].

2.2.1 Data Analytics

Medical research has historically been a data-driven discipline, with randomized clinical trials serving as the great standard in many ways. Due to recent developments in integrated electronic healthcare reports\medical, imaging, smart devices, clinical practice and medical sciences are increasingly evolving into big data focused environments. As a result, the healthcare sector as a patients, management, insurers, and policymakers will greatly benefit from emerging Big Data technology and, in particular, analytics. There are many challenges and criteria to developing advanced Big Data Analytics methods and techniques in healthcare. They shall include [9]:

Multi-modal Data
There is a perfect set of well-cured, structured and ordered data in data analytics, for example, as is also found in electronic health reports. However, the storage of unstructured data is a high proportion of health data. Any of them come in the form of real-time sensor readings, such as intensive care Electro Cardio Graph (ECG) measurements, medical clinical report text data, and natural language medical literature, imaging data, or customized medicine genomics data. In addition, the use of external data such as lifestyle information, e.g. disease control, geospatial data and epidemiological social media is becoming increasingly widespread. It is vital to obtain awareness from information. The goal should be to derive valuable information from these heterogeneous data, to make it available to clinicians and to incorporate expertise into the clinical history of patients.

Complex Background Knowledge
Medical knowledge must explain very complex phenomena using multi-level health information on medical care and procedures, lifestyle knowledge, and an overwhelming amount of accessible medical resources in the literature or trial archives. Medical data generally comes with complicated metadata which must be taken into consideration in order to view data optimally, draw conclusions, define logical explanations, and explain clinical decisions.

Highly Qualified End-Users
Highly trained end-users such as physicians, clinical analysts and bio-informatics, they still have a strong responsibility, which insists on high levels of consistency of analytical methods before placing their faith in patient treatment. The ideal analytical approach should however, to the extent possible, generate understandable patterns in order to encourage cross-checking of outcomes and to allow confidence in solutions. It should also allow expert-driven analytics to be controlled by an expert.

Privacy
The European commission, medical data is extremely classified information that is subject to strict legal protection. An adequate regulatory mechanism to allow the study of such data, as well as the creation of adequate private information computational tools to enforce this process, are essential for the realistic applicability and effect of data-driven medicine and health care.

Supporting Complex Decision
Supporting complex decision-making: image data processing, pathology, intensive care monitoring, or multi-morbidity treatment are examples of ways in which noisy data, in complex cases, and potentially missing information, must be used to make medical decisions. It should be assured that neither humans nor algorithms can always have an optimal solution, but they can need to take critical decisions or determine alternatives in a short period of time. Smart assistants for patients who use smartphones and new wearable systems and sensor technology to help patients monitor illnesses and lead healthier lives are another area of support for medical decision-making with potentially very large future effects.

2.2.2   Real-Time Analytics

Any time-critical healthcare applications need to take prompt action at a point where a particular event is detected in real-time analytics. Multiple sources of heterogeneous data provide the ability in real-time to obtain insights:

- Real-time analytics refers to analytics methods that can be used to evaluate and derive information from all available data and tools in real time before accessing the system.
- Instead of storing and processing data at some point in the future, data stream mining refers to the ability to analyze and process streaming data in the present state (or when it arrives). Complex case identification refers to the discovery and management of patterns over a variety of data sources, where patterns are high-level, semantically dense, and essentially made clear to the user [9].

2.2.3 Data Science Outlook in Healthcare Informatics

We accept that data analysis has a big role to play in the future of healthcare offerings. It is the primary capacity behind the development in precision medicine in the form of machine learning, widely accepted as a critically needed improvement in care. Although early attempts have proved difficult in offering diagnostic and treatment guidance, we expect data science to finally master that domain as well. It seems likely that most photographs of radiology and pathology will be processed by a computer at some point, taking into account rapid advances in data technology for imaging research. Speech and text recognition have also been used for activities such as patient contact and documentation of clinical records, and their use will grow.

In these health-care areas, the main challenge to data science is not whether the technologies will be capable of being successful enough, but rather to ensure that they are applied in daily clinical practice. Data science programs ought to be approved by authorities in order to have universal adoption, integrated into EHR systems, standardized to a fair degree that related goods work in the same manner, taught physicians, compensated by public or private payer organisations and updated in the field over time [6]. At the end of the day, these hurdles will be overcome, but they will take far longer to do so than it takes to mature the technology themselves.

2.2.4 Stages of Analytics

Analytics is not a one-off initiative; instead of a single endeavour, it is a continual, evolving way of operating that will change as demands and priorities move with the enterprise showing in Fig. 2.2. More sophisticated stages of research introduce potential for strategic modelling, such as forecasts, real-time insight and automatic decision-making, which can add tremendous benefit.

In order to predict potential target events, Predictive analytics analyzes historical data. This move towards forward-looking analytics from both a technology and business process viewpoint, it is a significant crossover for a company. Various mathematical and machine learning methods are used in predictive analysis and are built over time with the introduction of new evidence. Predictive analytics can be used to detect peaks in admissions by combining observational data from patient records with external metrics such as weather forecasts and social media to increase staff numbers. Prescriptive analytics combines predictive analytics by proposing a particular or a sequence of acts based on the forecast. In prescriptive solutions, data techniques such as modelling and deep learning, and even some cognitive models, could be used. Based in the previous example, a prescriptive strategy will provide a forecast for peaks in admission and then suggest process or prioritization changes to shorten the duration of stay to confirm that many more patients as appropriate are handled by the staff. These guidelines may be based on specific business operations or, in the case of cognitive systems, prior techniques that have shown the best results.

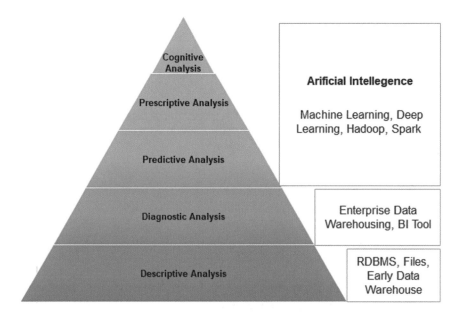

Fig. 2.2 Stages of analytics maturity and associated technologies

Data science methods such as artificial learning, deep learning and inference or logic systems are used in cognitive processing. It uses human-like analysis to auto-mate decisions or to offer observations and advice to improve human choices. This will help to give a full description of the patient's health, taking into account every-thing from the EMR records to the Computed Tomography (CT) scans to the patient's fitness tracking feed, as well as making proactive, real-time advice to the doctor on possible medication alternatives or risk factors, and providing patient updates with feedback about how to maintain their well-being [3].

2.2.5   Analytics Technologies

Picture it as constructing four complementary layers when developing an analytical environment, each with a range of innovations, depending on your own organizational requirements, legacy structures and priorities, and the form of analytics you require.

The Technology Layer
This is the basis for collecting, storing and preserving the data and running commer-cial and open source analytics. A variety of different systems, databases and applications can support a typical infrastructure layer [10].

The Data Layer

Internal pre-analytical repositories may also have made up the bulk of this sheet. This layer may take the form of a data lake (for example, based on the Cloudera Enterprise Data Hub) that incorporates multiple data sources into a single holistic environment, from EMR records to handwritten notes from clinicians to fitness tracker feeds, as today's data mix is more dynamic, dispersed, and unstructured. Several companies will provide several data systems, such as a relational database and a large data server, based on technologies such as Hadoop or NoSQL, side-by-side to satisfy various analytical and reporting criteria [10].

The Analytics Layer

This is the layer on which a majority of the enhancements can be added. There are various open source and business products available, with new implementations being launched on a regular basis. Technology engineering may be relatively new to some businesses, but there are numerous ways to innovate in the area of data processing. A layer of analytics should support a wide variety of algorithms [10]. Three of the most popular approaches used in data modelling are regression, sorting, and clustering algorithms. Most analytics systems can support the algorithm forms, as well as a few others to meet various needs.

The Applications Layer

The visualization of predictive model outcomes is assisted by this layer. Open source or commercial software offers customized analytics tools to support the individual cases and workflows of usage. Give close attention to how the effects of predictive models can be transmitted back to clinical stakeholders. When determining the best way to visualize and achieve outcomes, it is strongly recommended to engage a cross-functional team. Such questions that should be answered here are:

- What data in a pull vs. push system should be delivered? Should findings like the EMR or a new application be incorporated into an existing application?
- What details does a health worker need to be displayed? How do you calibrate outcomes in order to optimize signal vs. noise?
- How is it possible to capture data on the results of the model, either negatively or positively, in order to improve the model over time?

These layers allow you to take advantage of both the existing data management systems and emerging technology. Additional technology such as AI and efficiency or compliance solutions may be applied across the whole stack to drive insights and enhance data security [10].

2.3 Predictive Analytics

Predictive analytics helps assess what is extremely likely to happen in the future using modelling and forecasting techniques. These forecasts will then be used by

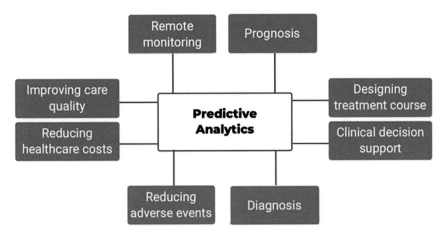

Fig. 2.3 The role of data science, predictive analysis, ML, AI in medical information

doctors, researchers, medical specialty societies, pharmaceutical firms, and any other healthcare stakeholder to provide the best possible treatment for individual patients [11]. Combining these new datasets with the latest epidemiology and clinical medicine sciences enables us to speed up progress in understanding the interactions between environmental factors and human biology, eventually leading to better clinical pathway reengineering and genuinely personalized treatment. Various role of predictive analysis are showing in Fig. 2.3.

2.3.1 Future of Predictive Analytics

Predictive analytics will become both more popular and more precise as we amass more and more data [12, 13]. Many predictive models currently use conventional statistical approaches, such as logistic regression, which are beneficial and can provide informative outcomes. Data science and machine learning techniques such as random forests, however, may provide more detailed predictions when properly applied. Ultimately, predictive analytics can take advantage of deep learning algorithms that can allow greater use of vast and complex data sets as more feature-rich data is gathered and as the collection process itself improves.

A machine learning-based approach will, on the other hand, require the radiologist to first extract all the features from the image. Deep learning simplifies the process by automatically detecting all the characteristics, without the radiologist needing extra work. Simply put, in healthcare, big data and predictive analytics go hand in hand. More data implies better predictions. Additionally, to address its limitations, the field of predictive analytics can progress. One current downside is that predictive analytics may not provide insight into what may happen after an operation or other improvement, which can be frustrating for researchers and clinicians who want to understand how patients may suffer after a new treatment or as a result of a new hospital procedure [10, 14]. We believe that predictive analytics will step beyond this hurdle, enabling researchers to forecast the future in a far more detailed and holistic manner. The vast leaps in computer processing power that make chewing through complicated algorithms possible would also be able to benefit from predictive analytics.

2.3.2   Reliability in Analytics

Often crucial in medical decision-making, often literally life or death-decisions must be reached under time constraints and under difficult and uncertain situations, if the right decision is not taken, with potentially serious mistakes [15]. Although recognizing that a data-driven method cannot be 100% reliable, and also understanding that neither doctor is necessarily right, very high expectations for medical data analysis are expected. Output measurement and management are also of vital significance. This is not only a basic ethical duty, but also an unaddressed accountability and protection issue that hinders the introduction of modern smart solutions into clinical practice. Many of the change would be based on this layer. There are various open source and commercial software available, with new implementations being published on a regular basis. Technology engineering may be new to some businesses, but there are also many possibilities for data processing innovation. A layer of analytics should be able to handle several different kinds of algorithms [10, 16]. Three of the most popular algorithms used in predictive analytics are regression, sorting, and clustering. Most analytics systems can support the algorithm styles, as well as a variety of others to meet various requirements.

2.4   Conclusion

Machine learning has been used by today's healthcare industry to achieve competitive advantage by rising productivity and reducing costs. With healthcare data the rapidly, data science will obviously work with you to help turn the stacks of information contained in electronic medical records, diagnostic information, and information on medical claims into cutting-edge insights and forecasts customized to your healthcare application. This chapter offers a general overview of personalized healthcare that affects the benefits of data science and methods of predictive analysis. It offers a comprehensive approach to facilitating the rapid growth, handling and study of medical data. There is also a need to monitor health care data, which is increasing at a high pace from time to time and on a larger scale with lots of inconsistent data sources, in order to produce more effective outcomes from healthcare. To exchange data between laboratories, hospital networks, and clinical centres, a distributed system should be arranged.

References

1. J. Kaur, K.S. Mann, HealthCare platform for real time, predictive and prescriptive analytics using reactive programming, in *10th International Conference on Computer and Electrical Engineering*, IOP Conf. Series: J. Phys.: Conf. Series 933, 012010 (2018). https://doi.org/10.1088/1742-6596/933/1/012010
2. P. Nieminen, Applications of medical informatics and data analysis methods. MDPI, Appl. Sci. **10**, 7359 (2020)
3. A. Bartley, Predictive Analytics in Healthcare, white paper—Healthcare Predictive Analytics, © Intel Corporation, Printed in USA 0917/FP/CAT/PDF 336536-001EN
4. https://www.cdc.gov/nchs/fastats/electronic-medical-records.htm
5. P. Desikan, R. Khare, J. Srivastava, R. Kaplan, J. Ghosh, L. Liu, V. Gopal, Predictive modeling in healthcare: challenges and opportunities. IEEE Life Sci. (2013)
6. S. Sinhasane, 14 Potential Use Cases of Data Science in Healthcare, https://mobisoftinfotech.com/resources/, 27 Mar 2019
7. H. Asri, H. Mousannif, H. Al Moatassime, T. Noel, Big data in healthcare: challenges and opportunities. Proc. Int. Conf. Cloud Comput. Technol. Appl. CloudTech (2015)
8. S. Sinhasane, https://mobisoftinfotech.com/resources/blog/data-science-in-healthcare-use-cases (2019)
9. P.J. Scott, R. Dunscombe, D. Evans, J.C. Wyatt, M. Mukherjee, Learning health systems need to bridge the 'two cultures' of clinical informatics and data science. J. Innov. Health Inform. **25**(2) (2018)
10. M. Ojha, K. Mathur, Proposed application of big data analytics in healthcare at Maharaja Yeshwantrao Hospital, in *3rd MEC International Conference on Big Data and Smart City (ICBDSC)*, 2016, pp. 1–7
11. C. Birkmeye, What Is Predictive Analytics and Why Is It Important? Healthcare Analytics, ArborMetrix (2020)
12. G. Palem, The Practice of Predictive Analytics in Healthcare, https://www.researchgate.net/publication/, 236336250 (2013)
13. A. Kankanhalli, J. Hahn, S. Tan, G. Gao, Big data and analytics in healthcare: introduction to the special section. Inf. Syst. Front. **18**(2), 233–235 (2016)
14. BDV, TF7 Healthcare subgroup, Big Data Technologies in Healthcare: Needs, opportunities and challenges (2016)
15. R. Ding, M.L. McCarthy, J. Lee, J.S. Desmond, S.L. Zeger, D. Aronsky, Predicting emergency department length of stay using quantile regression, in *2009 International Conference on Management and Service Science*, vol. 45, no. 2 (2009), pp. 1–4
16. W. Raghupathi, V. Raghupathi, Big data analytics in healthcare: promise and potential. Heal. Inf. Sci. Syst. **2**(1), 3 (2014)

Chapter 3
Eminent Role of Machine Learning in the Healthcare Data Management

Abstract The large quantities of data that can be produced in the medical sector. Each healthcare institution has its own patient records that include important details. When correctly evaluated, the healthcare domain will produce value from this data. A critical step necessary for the learning and application of clinical medicine is to bring medical informatics into the broad scope of medical education. Current main research areas can be categorized according to the organisation, introduction, and assessment of health information systems, the representation of medical expertise, and the study and interpretation of underlying signals and evidence. Machine learning has become really popular in the last few decades, and different methods of machine learning have been developed. It concentrates on the analyzing, developing, designing and implementing of techniques. The algorithms for machine learning use a well-defined learning method that best fits the purpose of the medical data analytics. Simple principles of the healthcare sector and machine learning will be defined in this study. The chapter shows how data analytics and machine learning can assist in the healthcare process, also posing certain obstacles, possibilities that need to be explored in order to achieve successful analytics in healthcare diagnosis.

Keywords Healthcare data · Data science · Machine learning · Medical informatics

3.1 Introduction

If we begin to promote the digitization of medical records, vast amounts of patient data are becoming readily accessible, both in terms of patient data given and medical outcomes produced by advanced equipment. A common consequence of this knowledge revolution is that the overwhelming challenge of processing and understanding the data is facing us. It is not only overwhelming to make sense of such a vast corpus of data; it is also impractical to use only manual instruments and techniques that can be a very slow and repetitive operation. In order to better interpret data, there is a desperate need for data-driven computer science methods, also referred

N. Thi Dieu Linh and Z. (Joan). Lu, *Data Science and Medical Informatics in Healthcare Technologies*, SpringerBriefs in Forensic and Medical Bioinformatics, https://doi.org/10.1007/978-981-16-3029-3_3

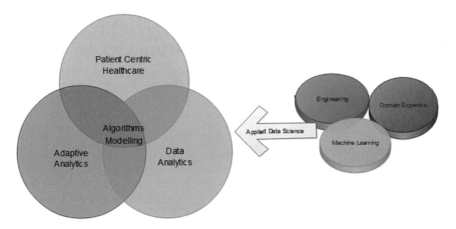

Fig. 3.1 Research frameworks for applied data science in patient-centric healthcare

to as data science or data analytics. In order to extract important clinical knowledge that can help patients and physicians make better decisions, these methods can be used to evaluate medical records. Today, in order to better interpret medical evidence, both industry and academia are beginning to make significant investments in the implementation of data science technology. Machine Learning (ML) is really the fastest-growing field of computer science, and medical informatics is one of the most challenging application problems, with potential benefits in better medical diagnosis, health analysis, and pharmaceutical growth. Successful machine learning for medical informatics, on the other hand, necessitates a concerted effort, fostering integrative research among both experts from various disciplines, from data science to visualization. Data science will have an important role to play in the coming years, with the exponential increase in the volume of data produced in medicine [1]. The data analytics systems in healthcare within applied data science context as specified above and in Fig. 3.1.

The study focuses on incorporating evidence and integrated information from a large body of research that could be able to leverage to promote future research. In order to establish and personalize early preventive and intervention initiatives and to promote access and exchange of testing protocols, records, metadata, and specimens, such investigations would implement data analytics in order to encourage cooperation, ensure reproducibility and validation of findings, and speed translation. The research on emerging patterns focuses mainly on four topics. The first covers connectivity, big data support systems and the expansion of data archives to facilitate direct access to integrated diverse biomedical resources and healthcare data. This study highlights obstacles, approaches to privacy preservation, and legal concerns for using human genomic data for confidential individual information. The second deals with the extraction and productive and creative use of information hidden in immense data volumes. The third theme reflects on the advancement of customized healthcare predictive analysis and modelling methods. In establishing predictive foundations of customized health care, big data analytics using a number of computer leaning methodologies play a key role. While training efforts and formal curricula have been around for more than a decade, a large skills gap continues to exist [2]

3.2 Machine Learning in Healthcare

The key goal of applied data science is to enhance, specifically, the physical world surrounding us in search of optimal social effects. In the areas of healthcare, defence, industry, education and social networks, as the use of big data becomes more widespread, academics have started to explore how data from these contexts can be properly processed, analyzed and mined. Note that applied data science analysis, in comparison to fundamental data science, mainly focuses on the implementation of machine learning techniques to address difficult problems in the everyday activities of domain experts by designing specialized computing systems that have an accessible and effective end-user environment in which machine learning or computational techniques can be implemented. In other words, it is not a primary goal of applied data science to build in a better way new computational and machine learning approaches for doing data science.

However, if it is not possible to adapt current machine learning techniques, this will cause further computational data science studies to establish the requisite methods for solving the issue at present. In addition, a specific increase in exposure is observed to such specialized software applications in the areas of healthcare, defence, industry, education, and social networks. These innovations seek to enhance the quality of work for doctors, patients, entrepreneurs, and educators in their everyday activities. Clinical threats, financial crises, and educational problems can also be minimized by innovative structures for applied data science. At the very same time, doctors, customers, entrepreneurs, and students would be part of the process, with more details directly transmitted to their smart phones. To provide a good service and dynamic recommendations to enhance the quality of life in any aspect and reduce risks, they can have more details. In other words, integrated data science will provide encouragement for doctors, patients, entrepreneurs and students, growing incentive for usage and, eventually, data creation, in turn [3].

3.2.1 Machine Learning in Medical Field

Machine learning has been very common in the last few decades and different methods of machine learning have been produced. In contrast to the most widely implemented machine learning algorithms, this section would summarize the core principles of machine learning. Machine learning is an Artificial Intelligence (AI) area of research that encourages computers to be smarter without human intervention, i.e., it allows machines the potential to understand using past observations and interactions on their own. It focuses on the planning, study, creation and application of approaches that can access and use knowledge to learn on their own.

Today, in diverse areas such as telecommunications, banking, search engines, medical sciences, machine learning is commonly adapted. Machine learning in the medical field can enable very difficult and time-consuming assignments. It is thus implemented in different fields of pharmacy.

Disease Diagnosis/Identification
One primary motivation through which the medical profession will benefit to a great degree is the detection of diseases. In the medical industry, machine learning can be introduced to help doctors save time by identifying diseases in their initial stages. In research on machine learning techniques cancer, diabetes detection, brain tumours is a widely studied field. Current trials have focused on cancer identification in order to promote the early study of cancer diagnosis and disease detection.

Drug Discovery
IBM and Google began other health ventures by applying machine learning to find medications in their early days. By minimizing the expense and time of the drug development process, these ventures surpass the boundaries of drug research, with conventional drug discovery taking years to produce only one new drug.

Healthcare Data Analytics
Many machine learning models are used for medical data processing; analytics can become very useful and interesting in better understanding disease processes, predicting diseases, and even preventing diseases. Using machine learning rather than spending hours or even days on data processing might allow practitioners save lives by saving time. There are so many more areas where machine learning is efficient, and the explanations for machine learning can never be exhausted.

3.3   Healthcare Data Management and Data Infrastructure

The medical records are extremely complicated. They are made up of unorganized, organized, and processed information. A particular entity's traditional healthcare data archives could contain 3.5 GB of data, while advanced deep-phenotyping assessment methods including high-content imaging and genomics could generate an additional 120 GB of data [4]. Data collection can be complicated by the diversity of records and the distribution of information throughout different channels. As a result, as seen in Fig. 3.2, modernizing the fundamental infrastructures for data collection, acquisition, and management is a top priority. Usual procedure will call for data lake specifications (fundamental storage of broad native data sets), databases and Application Programming Interfaces (APIs) to serve different uses.

Access and retrieval of data are usually seen from the point of view of administrative demands, for instance for billing purposes, while the end user or patient is paying

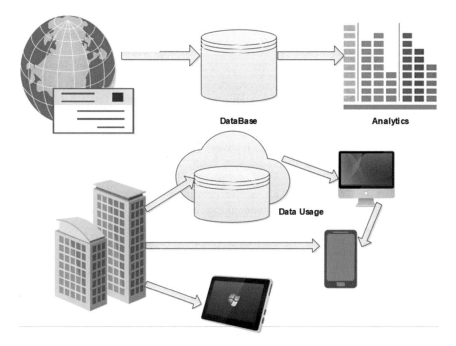

Fig. 3.2 Evolving concepts in data usage and analytics

less attention. In the history of medical records, we proposed that medical records should be readily searchable and conveniently available so that patients can consult for any word and immediately locate their associated documentary or pictures. This definition, reflecting how simple it is to communicate with resources like Google, also implies the use of consumer cantered technology to establish access to electronic medical records [4]. Genomics will also expand the conception of health and biomedical scientists who can use search engines to easily search for gene variants method that was used to facilitate the searchability of the non-coding genomes.

3.3.1   Healthcare Data Ownership and Portability

Health records are a unique electronic documentation. Unlike conventional natural properties, which can be controlled by one person at a time, they can be copied and disseminated easily. They are unique, non-depletive and replicable. But sometimes, these features can present particular difficulties in data quality management. Data portability is the freedom of consumers to monitor their data free mobility between alternative service providers and thereby facilitate free markets competition. However, data portability in the United States requires compromised health data security due to the restricted amount of individuals protected, liable for personal health safety and privacy [4]. Due to data control interests, the enormous complexity of the medical infrastructure and a lack of general protocols for information exchange, the disruption of data portability have become further exacerbated.

The adoption of standards is a key issue in data portability, and some of the active efforts available to communicate Electronic Health Records (EHRs), Digital Imaging and Communications in Medicine (DICOM), such as Health Level Seven (HL7) international and Fast Healthcare Interoperability Resources (FHIR) [4]. Importantly we should not explore the relevant obligation for data management. A new study discussed the liability concerns in the area of genomics. We should not even speak about the ethical challenges where patient knowledge is a commodity and qualified machine learning models are used without permission. As competitors can use reverse engineering models to disclose sensitive details from participants in the training dataset, there is a chance of confidential data being leaked [4]. We believe that an informing consent process or educational solution should be used to educate the community about some of these affected legal problems of privacy.

3.3.2 Data Science and Machine Learning Applications in Healthcare

Neuro-imaging is one of the most well-known uses of cluster analysis in the medical world. Advanced Magnetic Resonance Imaging (MRI) approaches allow for ground-breaking insights into the brain's complex mechanisms. It was also used for scientific trials where an immense volume of knowledge has to be analyzed to identify patterns that explain the healthy brain's structure and function and its disease-related alternatives. For neuro-imaging applications such as segmentation of fibre tracks and lesions, some clustering approaches are used, as well as methods that can work with multimodal image images. In fact, clustering is an important tool that can assist with diagnostic research. Some of the healthcare applications are explained here and some important listed in Table 3.1.

Disease Monitoring and Prevention
Data scientists use strong statistical computational methods for the early identification of chronic diseases. In certain severe circumstances, there are situations where viruses are not caught at an early stage due to negligibility [5]. This appears to be particularly harmful not only to the welfare of the patient, but also to the economic costs. As the disease progresses, it also raises the cost of treating it. Therefore, in order to maximize economic expenditure on healthcare, data science plays a significant role. Through looking at all these healthcare uses of data technology, we might conclude that data science is one of human beings' great inventions. So, we believe that healthcare has multiple uses in data science. Data analysis has been used extensively by the medicine and healthcare industries to change patient's lives and forecast illnesses at an early stage. In addition, with improvements in medical image processing, it is possible for doctors to recognize microscopic tumours that may

Table 3.1 Data science and ML applications and technology adoption

S. No.	Applications	Reason for Technology Adoption
1	Detection of Frauds	Need to address increasingly payment fraud attempts and complex service
2	Robot supported surgery	Technological advances in robotic solutions for more types of surgery
3	Virtual attention support	Hospital labour shortages are putting more strain on the system
4	Dosage inaccuracy reduction	Medical inaccuracies are common, and they result in monetary penalties
5	Organizational workflow	Integration of current application networks is made easier
6	Clinical assessment contribution	The patent cliff: a plethora of data: a results-oriented approach
7	Associated machines	Increase in the number of wired computers and devices
8	Programmed image diagnosis	Greater trust in AI technologies due to storage space
9	Preliminary diagnosis	To improve consistency, interoperability data architecture was developed
10	Cyber security	Increased responsibility to secure patient records as a result of data breaches

otherwise be impossible to spot. Therefore, computer science in wide respects has revolutionized healthcare and the medical sector.

Research of Medicines

If the population of the planet increases, every now and then there are several problems of a human body arising. This may be attributed to a lack of enough health, fear, pollution, physical diseases, etc. Now, discovering drugs or vaccines for diseases in a short period has become a problem for medical research institutes. Since researchers have to consider the properties of the causative agent in order to find a formula for a drug, it may take millions of test cases to do this. Then, the researchers have to run further experiments on the formula after discovering a formula. It is possible to process data from millions of test cases within months or hours. It helps to determine the drug's efficacy by data collection. Therefore, it is possible to launch a successfully tested vaccine or drug in less than a year. With the assistance of data science and machine learning, this is all feasible. Both also revolutionized the areas of medicinal drug discovery and development. First, we can see the data science framework in genomics [6].

Virtual Support

A perfect example of the use of data technology is the software which is developed with interactive assistance. Data scientists have developed extensive systems that give patients a customized experience. The diagnostic systems that use data science support a patient by evaluating the signs to classify the illness. The patient has to enter his/her symptoms only and the program will predict the patient's illness and condition. Precautions, prescription, and care needed as per the patient's condition will be suggested [6]. In addition, the program analyzes the patient's details and generates a checklist of the treatment processes to be pursued. Then, the patient is periodically informed of use. It aims to deter a negligence incident that may make the situation worse. For patients suffering from alzheimer's, anxiety, depression, and other neurological conditions, interactive support has often shown to be helpful. The care of these patients becomes productive when the request frequently notifies them of the requested steps being taken. Proper medicine, fitness, and dietary consumption are included in those steps.

Data Governance and Data Administration
The potential for improved handling of records is immense. Moving for greater use of open practices and better top-level exchange of knowledge offers actionable transparency into the activity of the health service. Machine learning would encourage physicians to be more compassionate and offer quality treatment. Data processing is all about making data readily available to persons in the healthcare sector who work [6]. As the essence of the health sector is risk-entailing, to determine the actual situation and future consequences, data crunching must be ultra-cautious. Furthermore, healthcare data analytics should stay up-to-date, complete, and profound.

Genetics/Genomics—Treatment Personalization
If it's multiple ways of genomic profiling sequencing or something else, this gives a fresh glimpse at the genomics field as new innovations come along. With massive volumes of information today, genetic information is now generated faster than it can be processed or applied. Part of this is because the strategies for data structuring lag significantly behind improving the capacity to collect knowledge. Data science for healthcare is a positive idea, so you need to be able to make use of it [6].

3.3.3 Machine Learning and Predictive Analytics

Healthcare data analytics solutions in healthcare exploit the data boom to obtain insights and make better-informed choices as well as to increase the quality of health care and decrease costs by allowing more preventive and tailored care. Analytics have proved to be beneficial here too. A new Intel commissioned report from the International Institute for Analytics finds that it is used by the top performers in healthcare analytics to further boost patient participation, population wellbeing, and quality of treatment and business processes, sectors that directly map to the quadruple targets. However, understanding where to begin can be tricky for those who are not already fluent in analytics. Advanced computational approaches such as machine learning and data science offer ground-breaking insights and great breakthrough opportunities, but they can also be nuanced and overwhelming. The method of learning from past evidence to make assumptions about the future is predictive analysis. Predictive analytics would allow the right options to be made for health care, enabling care to be tailored for each client. The wheel is not being reinvented by predictive analytics. This is what doctors have been doing on a broader scale. Our ability to better assess, aggregate, and make sense of historically difficult-to-obtain or non-existent mental, psychosocial and biometric knowledge has changed. In healthcare data analytics, examples of focused fields include:

Evidence-based medicine. In which a range of statistics are combined and evaluated to align effects of treatment, predict patients at risk of infection or readmission, and deliver more appropriate care.

Device/remote monitoring and mobile health. Where we collect and interpret real-time data for security monitoring and adverse event prediction from in-hospital and in-home applications.

Patient profile analytics. Where we apply analytics to patient accounts to identify patients who would benefit from supportive treatment or lifestyle changes; and

Genomic analytics. Where gene processing is done more accurately and cost-effectively. Genomic analysis is part of the daily decision-making process for medical treatment. It will help to optimize treatment, save lives, and decrease costs by finding connections and recognizing patterns and trends within the data.

The complexities of recording, preserving, scanning, exchanging, and evaluating this massive volume of information includes:

- Inferring information from diverse origins of heterogeneous patients,
- Leveraging associations of patient/data between documents,
- Extracting from clinical data notes information and observations,
- To process vast quantities of medical imaging data effectively and to extract potentially valuable information and biomarkers,
- Interpreting and integrating genomic data with normal clinical data, and
- Collecting the interpersonal knowledge of the patient through multiple sensors their diverse social experiences and messages [7].

3.4 Healthcare Informatics

Health informatics is concerned with information management that allows for the effective collection of data using technical tools in order to enhance medical knowledge and facilitate the quality of medical care to patients. Medical informatics' goal is to ensure that critical patient medical information is accessible at the precise time and place needed to make medical decisions. Health informatics also deals with the processing of patient data for research and education. Three papers in this scientific literature suggest therapeutic decision-making implementations.

Daniel Clavel and his co-authors [8] suggest a decision-support system for coordinating and ordering future surgeries. Their research has the potential to reduce the healthcare sector's planning load, which is extremely labor-intensive. In the framework for decision support, a heuristic algorithm is proposed and used. Various aspects are implemented in a software tool with a friendly user interface. It shows and analyzes a simulation comparison of scheduling done using the framework outlined in this paper versus other methods. Furthermore, in one hospital environment, the effect of the software tool on the reliability and consistency of surgical facilities is studied.

Joaquín Rodríguez, Gilberto Ochoa-Ruiz, and Christian Mata presented a new Graphical User Interface (GUI) method based on semi-automated prostate segmentation in a complete and comprehensive manner in their article, A Prostate MRI segmentation tool based on active contour models using a gradient vector flow [8]. The aim is to promote the time-consuming method of segmentation used in clinical practice for annotating images. The authors present an experimental case to support the efficiency of their process.

Hernandez-Ordonez and colleagues' research, Medical Assistant Smartphone Application for Diabetes Treatment by Simulating a Compartmental Model [8], is very interesting and innovative. The writers implement a type 1 diabetes assistant patient mobile phone service. The proposed solution is based on four computer models which use a parametric model to describe glucose-insulin-glucagon dynamics, as well as supplementary mechanisms to simulate aerobic activity, gastric glucose absorption by the stomach, and subcutaneous insulin absorption. Such advances are always welcome because diabetes has become an illness of humanity that affects a number of individuals every year. For the reasons stated, research in healthcare analytics is shifting to exploit machine learning methods:

Latest Types of Data
Medicine is progressing towards customized mentoring and care through scientific advancements in neuroscience, mapping, signal analysis, and Radio Frequency Identification (RFID), to name a few. This has created a number of unorthodox ways of knowledge as well. There is also a need for machine learning to scale up to the spectrum of types of data.

The Spectrum of Statistical Research with Respect to Data
Individually directed statistical learning is a process. It is driven by a series of predefined hypotheses and is based on the confirmation of a fixed hypothesis. In comparison, general population projections have been focused on mathematical analysis. Machine learning, on the other hand, is used to generate hypotheses. It is more inquisitive and based on fewer hypotheses. However, the only difference between mathematical analysis and machine learning is that machine learning is motivated by data.

The Scalability of Processes
With data growth approaching an exponential pace, algorithms and techniques are required that can leverage the data produced and provide forecasts that can scale up

to data shifts, as well as uncover unknown and non-trivial observations that cannot be manually performed [9].

3.4.1 Machine Learning Approaches for Medical Informatics

Machine learning provides a broad variety of methods to learning that can be picked from the data to capture hidden patterns. We categorize these approaches into three and give the following brief description of these categories:

Non-monitored Methods
Machine learning's unsupervised approaches are those which discover secret data patterns or trends. Such methods aim to define key features that drive distinction between samples of data. These methods are often referred to as clustering and are prominently used in signal processing systems. Spectral clustering, Gaussian mixture simulations, K-means, fuzzy clustering are some of the frequently referenced unsupervised methods. However, since these methods are subject to fixed thresholds, they suffer from a bottleneck.

Supervised Approaches
The aim of supervised learning methods is to specify specific sets of rules which can be used to distinguish between samples from various classes. For example, Decision Trees (DT) is a supervised approach to learning that is simple to understand and implement. In contrast to unsupervised methods, supervised approaches are used to construct models. These techniques use a pre-processed training collection of samples to create a model, with each sample in the classification algorithm having a particular class name.

Ensemble or Hybrid Approaches
The hybrid or ensemble methods are based on the premise that effective discriminatory rules can be created by a combination of several single models. In addition, each of the single models has its strengths and intrinsic drawbacks that can be solved in the ensemble by other models. However, integrating multiple models to solve the drawbacks of a single model can lead to over-fitting problems.

3.5   Challenges in Healthcare Data Analytics in Healthcare

The development of advanced tools and techniques for data analytics in healthcare is fraught with difficulties. Among them are [10]:

Multimodal Data
In data processing, for example, there is an ideal array of structured and organized material, as seen in electronic health records. However, a substantial number of

patient reports are made up of unstructured files [11]. Many of it is in the type of actual sensed data, such as ECG measures in intensive care, natural language medical literature, text data from physician clinical reports genomics data or personalized medicine image data. In addition, it is becoming more popular to use external data such as lifestyle information, e.g. for disease control, or geospatial data and epidemiological social media. Gaining insights from the information is vital. The aim should be to gain useful information by multimodal learning from such heterogeneous data, make the lessons from such integrated information accessible to clinicians and integrate expertise into patients' clinical history.

Complex Background Knowledge
Medical evidence must clarify very complex phenomena, ranging from multi-level patient reports on medical conditions and medications, nutrition, and evidence to the vast amount of available medical knowledge in testing, bio banks, and study repositories [12]. As a result, medical data also comes with nuanced metadata that must be considered in order to efficiently analyze the data, locate logical interpretations, reach conclusions, and support treatment decisions.

Explainable Trustworthy Models
End users with medical analytical instruments, such as surgeons, healthcare analysts and bioinformaticians, are highly trained [13]. They still have a strong obligation, which is focused on high standards of the efficiency of diagnostic instruments before putting their confidence in patient care. Therefore, as far as possible, an optimal analytical method should produce understandable patterns in order to allow outcomes to be cross-checked and to allow confidence in the solutions. This should also allow expert-driven self-service analytics to encourage the analytics process to be managed by the expert.

Supporting Complex Decision
Visual feedback processing, multi-morbidity treatment, critical care tracking and pathology are only a few examples of how noisy results, potentially unreliable knowledge and complex situations would be used to make such decisions [14, 15]. While neither humans nor algorithms are guaranteed to have the right solution, they may be forced to make crucial decisions or define alternatives in a limited period of time. Another area of medical decision support with potentially large future implications is smart assistants for patients who use smart phones, new wearable gadgets, and sensor systems to help patients monitor conditions and lead healthier lives.

Privacy
Patient data is highly sensitive material that is subject to stringent legal safeguards at the European level. An effective regulatory mechanism to allow the analysis of such data, as well as the provision of sufficient privacy-preserving analytical tools to implement this framework, are essential for the practical applicability and impact of data-driven medicine and healthcare [16].

Approaches for tackling data analytics in the light of the above-mentioned problems are presented as follows:

Advanced Machine Learning and Reinforcement Learning

Reinforcement learning is a modern, highly promising, sophisticated machine learning methodology with a trial-and-error paradigm of learning purely from incentives or penalties. It has been successfully used in breakthrough technology.

Deep Learning

Deep learning is a term that corresponds to a range of machine learning algorithms that are built on interpretations of learning information (capturing highly nonlinear relationships of low-level unstructured input data to form high-level concepts). Deep learning algorithms have made significant progress in a number of areas where traditional machine learning techniques have struggled, machine translation, including speech recognition, computer vision (object recognition) etc.

Real-Time Analytics

Some time-critical healthcare applications need to take precautions right from the moment that a real incident is observed. The ability to extract insights in real time is given by several sources of heterogeneous data. There are many important, interconnected approaches:

- Real-time analytics applies to analytics strategies that, when they enter a framework, can interpret and extract information from all available data [17] and tools in real time.
- Instead of saving the data and extracting it at some time in the future, data stream mining refers to the ability to analyze and process streaming data in the moment.
- The identification and maintenance of patterns over multiple data sources [18] applies to dynamic event identification, where patterns are high-level, semantically rich and eventually rendered accessible to the user.

Understanding and Reliability in Analytics

Many important decisions, often involving life or death, must be taken in medical decision-making under time constraints and under complex and ambiguous situations, with the potential for serious consequences if the wrong decision is made. Although recognizing that a data-driven approach will never be 100% reliable, and accepting that neither doctor is necessarily right, medical implementations for data analytics are held to extremely high standards. It's often important to determine and track performance (for example, the consistency of data-driven systems). Understanding, particularly for complex optimization techniques that evolve over time from a large number of new data input, is a key characteristic of an empirical approach that inspires confidence in its practical implementation. Reliability has also been identified as a major difficulty, especially for complex learning systems that build up over time from a constant stream of new input data.

3.6   Conclusion

The significance to individuals and governments of healthcare and it's the cost to the economy have led to the rise of healthcare as a significant research subject field for business academics and other researchers. The use of ubiquitous computing will take advantage of both the efficiency of health services and the regulation of patient care costs. Basic concepts of the medical field and machine learning will be described in this chapter. We can illustrate how data mining will aid in the healthcare process. Data science and machine learning have been turned from intellectual curiosity into a broad field of healthcare and medical data processing in recent years. Abundant machine learning work has attracted interest in optimization science, inspired by large-scale applications that involve huge, high-dimensional data processing. This study illustrates that artificial learning and predictive processing have provided new methods for care practitioners to work with, new approaches to practice medical conditions. It also confirms that in the health care province, machine learning methods and strategies are definitive and used exclusively in the detection and prediction. In the medical industry, computer science and deep learning algorithms are widely adapted because of their remarkable ability to learn rapidly. In many fields of medical care, especially in medical data analytics, groundbreaking advances have been seen. However, some problems, mixed results, ever-changing evidence-based medicine and deceptive outliers also impact these approaches.

References

1. N.G. Maity, S. Das, Machine Learning for Improved Diagnosis and Prognosis in Healthcare, 978-1-5090-1613-6/17/$31.00 ©2017 IEEE
2. N.R. Adam, R. Wieder, D. Ghosh, Data science, learning, and applications to biomedical and health sciences, in *Issue: Data Science, Learning, and Applications to Biomedical and Health Sciences*, Ann. N.Y. Acad. Sci. 1387 (2017) 5–11 C 2017 New York Academy of Sciences
3. M. Spruit, M. Lytras, Applied data science in patient-centric healthcare. Telematics Inform. (2018). https://doi.org/10.1016/j.tele.2018.04.002
4. A. Telenti, X. Jiang, Treating medical data as a durable asset. NATure GeNeTics **52**, 1005–1010 (2020)
5. D. Delen, H. Demirkan, Data, information and analytics as services, © 2012 Elsevier, May 2012
6. M. Ojha, K. Mathur, Proposed application of big data analytics in healthcare at Maharaja Yeshwantrao Hospital, in *2016 3rd MEC International Conference on Big Data and Smart City (ICBDSC)*, 2016, pp. 1–7
7. National Institutes of Health. Big Data to Knowledge (BD2K). Accessed 12 Dec 2016. https://datascience.nih.gov/bd2k
8. P. Nieminen, Applications of medical informatics and data analysis methods, in *Medical Informatics and Data Analysis Research Group*, University of Oulu, 90014 Oulu, Finland. Appl. Sci. **10**(20), 7359 (2020)
9. P. Chowriappa, S. Dua, Y. Todorov, Introduction to machine learning in healthcare informatics, in *Machine Learning in Healthcare Informatics*, December 2014 Intelligent Systems Reference Library, vol. 56, pp. 1–23

10. S. Consoli, D.R. Recupero, M. Petkovic, Data Science for Healthcare Methodologies and Applications. https://doi.org/10.1007/978-3-030-05249-2 © Springer Nature Switzerland AG 2019

11. G. Palem, The Practice of Predictive Analytics in Healthcare, no. July, 2013

12. D.W. Bates, S. Saria, L. Ohno-Machado, A. Shah, G. Escobar, Big data in health care: using analytics to identify and manage high-risk and high-cost patients. Health Aff. **33**(7), 1123–1131 (2014)

13. R. Chauhan, R. Jangade, A robust model for big healthcare data analytics, in *2016 6th International Conference—Cloud System and Big Data Engineering (Confluence)*, 2016, pp. 221–225

14. R. Ding, M.L. McCarthy, J. Lee, J.S. Desmond, S.L. Zeger, D. Aronsky, Predicting emergency department length of stay using Quantile regression, in *2009 International Conference on Management and Service Science*, 2009, vol. 45, no. 2, pp. 1–4

15. P.J. Scott, R. Dunscombe, D. Evans, J.C. Wyatt, M. Mukherjee, Learning health systems need to bridge the 'two cultures' of clinical informatics and data science. J. Innov. Health Inform. **25**(2) (2018)

16. P. Nieminen, Applications of medical informatics and data analysis methods. MDPI, Appl. Sci. **10**, 7359 (2020)

17. B. Nithya, V. Ilango, Predictive analytics in health care using machine learning tools and techniques, in *International Conference on Intelligent Computing and Control Systems ICICCS* 2017

18. K. Gray, "Scitechnol Journals Press Releases" Biomedical Informatics uses computation to extract data from biological data, 06 Jan 2020

Chapter 4
Potential and Adoption of Data Science in the Healthcare Analytics

Abstract The creation and validation of clinical practice predictive models is just the initial step in the path towards mainstream adoption of predictions for real-time point-of-care. Adoption of healthcare analytics can occur at diverse levels, including medical error tracking and avoidance, data integration, predictive analysis and personalized modelling. Although substantial advancement and progress has been made from the perspective of data science and study, challenges and opportunities remain. Current main fields of study can be categorized according to the organisation, introduction, and assessment of health information systems, patient information representation, and analysis and interpretation of underlying signals and data. We should anticipate many shifts in future medical informatics science in view of the fluid existence of many of the driving factors behind advancement in knowledge management methods and their technology, developments in medicine and health care, and the constantly shifting demands, requirements and aspirations of human populations. This chapter will explain the relevance of the application of predictive analytics strategies focused on data science in healthcare. By way of intelligent process analysis and medical data mining, the device would be able to derive real time valuable information that aids in decision making and medical tracking.

Keywords Data science · Predictive analysis · Medical informative · Healthcare analysis

4.1 Introduction

As with the transformation of time and technological upgrades, there is a need to make structural reforms to health programs in order to maximize the quality, efficiency and viability of patient care. The strategic aim of value based healthcare is to ensure that everyone can make use of the health services required for their health and well-being. Focus on value-based treatment leads to an intensified emphasis on patient-cantered treatment. A doctor, clinics, and health insurers must collaborate with each other to customize treatment that is reliable, consistent in its implementation and billing, and assessed by concentrating on technology and healthcare systems on patient outcomes

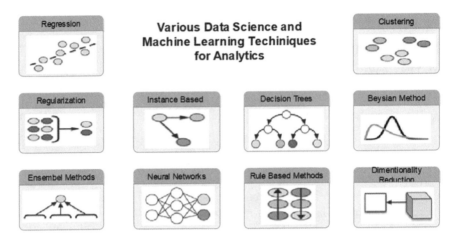

Fig. 4.1 Data science and machine learning techniques for analytics [3]

based on satisfaction of the patient. It was expected that Electronic Health Reports (EHRs) and comprehensive data processing by health care providers would increase the efficacy and quality of patient care [1]. Statistics research refers to the creation and implementation of instruments for planning, evaluating and interpreting observational medical studies. The creative use of statistical inference theory, a clear understanding of clinical and epidemiological testing issues and an understanding of the value of statistical software rely on the development of new statistical methods for medical applications [2] (Fig. 4.1).

In almost every area, data analytics has become increasingly relevant. Health care provides a wide variety of private and public data collection programs that provide multiple data bases. When health-care professionals have switched to EHRs, digital laboratory slides, videos, and high-resolution radiology photographs over the last century, the number of facts has grown exponentially. In health-care institutions' archives, terabytes of data of data are collected, and millions of data sets are transmitted from devices such as behavioural trackers and other ongoing screening systems. Healthcare digitization aims to create a wide variety of new data sets. The Electronic medical database is one of the most important examples of this. It is expected that data from genomics will expand substantially in the future as precision medicine is gradually incorporated into traditional clinical workflows. With the use of fitness workout and activity trackers and software apps, healthcare facilities produce a large volume of health data outside of the hospital setting. The introduction of health-related Internet of Things (IoT) software, as well as apps and other wellness technology, produces a huge volume of data on a regular basis. Healthcare companies have a tremendous potential to incorporate these disparate data sets and processes with emerging technology. In addition to the hospital's own archives, external information such as social networks or publicly accessible government statistics may be used to consider community health patterns. However, 94% of hospitals do not actually collect sufficient knowledge to perform effective public health analyzes [4].

4.1.1 Challenges

Big data analytics in healthcare comes with many challenges including privacy and security [5].

Privacy

As companies cooperate and exchange information to allow an automated EMR, privacy becomes critical. For the purposes of statistical analytics and demographic studies, privacy must be maintained when sharing information and maintaining much of the usefulness of aggregated data while adhering to privacy limits. When data from different sources is combined, the privacy-utility tradeoffs become much more important to consider, eventually leading to accidental effects or leaks.

Security

Data security is a top concern for health organisations, particularly in the wake of a string of high-profile breaches and hacks. Healthcare data is vulnerable to an apparently unlimited range of threats. In practice, these safeguards take the form of commonly agreed security procedures like using up-to-date anti-virus applications, firewall tuning, private data protection, and multi-factor authentication.

Analytics

In data processing and management, there are several problems resulting from missing, heterogeneous, inaccurate, or contradictory data. The selection of key data elements based on high utility value and the viability of collection are critical for effective data analytics. The challenges with working with vast quantities of future predictors and the rarity of many of the incidents of concern must also be resolved by such analytics.

Execution of Technology

The main hurdles to the acceptance and understanding of predictive modelling methods in health care can be analyzed at two levels, namely the adoption and usage of devices. The first is attributed to a lack of understanding of its usefulness and a lack of compliance with the strategic goals. Clinicians are incredibly busy, and little motivation has been provided to explore how analytics can make them more sensitive and efficient. Data access and sharing features are often limited by safety and sensitivity concerns associated with medical data. In challenging clinical workflows, processes, and settings, the second set of problems is consistent with real device use. When dealing with electronic medical records on a regular basis, physicians face a host of difficulties. While EMRs offer help for entering structured data, due to the shortage of time and system accessibility, clinicians frequently return to unstructured notes. This adds to problems in natural language interpretation and data errors.

Lack of Involvement of Data Scientists

For research and understanding, clinicians have historically focused heavily on biostatisticians. There is potential to implement approaches from large-scale data analytics applications in other fields as data processing capabilities evolve and large volumes of data are generated. Therefore, exploiting the expertise of data scientists when designing analytical solutions is increasingly necessary. In healthcare services itself, with the possible exception of the payers, the acceptance and implementation of certain expertise has been incremental, although there is a growing understanding of the need.

4.1.2 Possibilities

Compared to other sectors, such as finance and banking, the issues mentioned above, along with other lawful and regulatory restrictions, make healthcare a late adopter of technology. Although several technological problems are of concern, the major possibilities include [6].

Research Opportunities

It would be important to apply domain expertise and real life information to resolve data quality challenges to further enhance the efficacy of predictive modelling follow-up efforts. It would be important to pick function strategies, since much of the data in healthcare is very large. In integrating evidence from multiple sources, smart ensemble approaches can play a crucial role. Finally, for effective teamwork and for the convergence of data from multiple sources, privacy-aware and knowledge-preserving data sharing strategies are important. The harmonization of data components through data processing schemes is one of the most critical problems. It will provide new avenues for epidemiological studies to achieve consensus about what is calculated. What is calculated in the clinical practice arena should determine what issues get clinical treatment. In their workflow, meeting the needs of clinicians: Strategies should concentrate on making processes smarter and simpler for doctors to work with. For example, a method that summarizes key points in a text format and answers clinicians' concerns when looking at medical records will encourage physicians to focus on patient care rather than data analysis and data analysis. Technology deployment will be driven by usability and efficiency.

Interdisciplinary Design Teams

While there is a strong consensus on the need for physicians and data scientists to work together and work together to create and build effective technical solutions, a more coherent and cohesive interdisciplinary team of physicians, data scientists, biostatisticians, epidemiologists, policy makers, legal experts, etc. is required. Otherwise, most healthcare programs will ultimately be built in a narrow context that does not offer effective alternatives, leading to frustration and loss of confidence in the success of those systems [3].

4.2 The Utility of Data Science in Healthcare

Without a doubt Artificial Intelligence (AI) and Machine Learning (ML) have been hot topics in all fields, including healthcare. Companies are racing to stock up on data scientists, big and small, but are data scientists alone adequate to create an effective healthcare data science practice? Data scientists are, without a doubt, essential to construct models. But you need a whole network of support functions to grow and maintain the team as you deal with healthcare and human data [7]. Big data in healthcare involves the vast volumes of data that have been made available to healthcare providers since the advent of digitalisation in the sector. Systematic analysis of these data sets will provide actionable information to help to take better decisions about health care issues. This aims to develop a systematic and balanced view of patients, clients and physicians.

4.2.1 Why Healthcare Analytics?

Data collection, data sharing, and data analysis are three cycles of data mining that have slowed healthcare in the United States and other parts of the world. To date, the processing and dissemination of data waves, which are marked by the urgent introduction of EHRs and the exchange of health information, have had little effect on healthcare quality and expense. In certain cases, the constant emphasis on data has led to an over-focus on the EHR, resulting in provider burnout and time and resources diverted from patients. Despite the recent buzz around big data being the next big thing in other markets, we are only just getting started in healthcare with the statistical technologies that will help quality assurance and cost-cutting measures across the board. Healthcare analysis is the organized use of data to create practical information. The true potential of analytics is to turn healthcare into a data-driven environment powered by world-class analytics platforms [8].

4.2.2 The Healthcare Analytics Adoption Model

Health data and analytics can be daunting and frustrating without a vision and a goal-oriented structure. When the healthcare market lacked a robust analytics model that met the particular demands of health data, a group of cross-industry healthcare veterans came up with the healthcare analytics adoption model. Throughout their analytical journey, health institutions should turn to the model as it offers comprehensive guidelines on the classification of analytical capability classes and provides standardized sequencing within the health system for the application of analytics. For health systems, any kind of predictive model is essential because the correct model can pave the groundwork for a viable, competitive analytics approach that can handle more diverse data needs in the future.

4.2.3   The Nine Levels of the Analytics Adoption Model [8]

Levels of the data analytics adoption model is describe here in Fig. 4.2.

Level 0—Fragmented Point Solutions

- Fragmented Point Solutions: inefficient, contrasting versions of truth.
- In order to address unique analytical demands as they emerge, vendor-based and internally developed software are used.

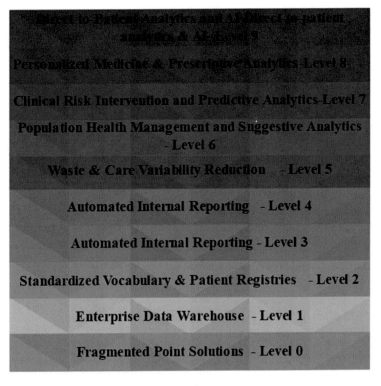

Fig. 4.2 Levels of the analytics adoption model [8]

- Highly fragmented point solutions that are neither co-located nor otherwise architecturally significant incorporated in a data warehouse.
- Multiple overlapping data content leads to contradictory explanations of empiric evidence.
- The results are labour-intensive and inconsistent.

Level 1—Enterprise Data Warehouse

- Corporate Data Warehouse Data and Knowledge Base:
- The following data are at least co-located in a single data warehouse, geographically or hosted: Health Information Management Systems Society (HIMSS), EMR, sales period, economical, costing, supply chain, and patient experience.
- The archive of searchable metadata is open to the enterprise.
- Information content includes insurance claims, where necessary.
- After one month of changes to the source computer, the data warehouse is updated.
- Data management takes place in terms of the data consistency of the source systems.

Level 2—Standardized Vocabulary and Patient Registries

- Structured Terminology and Patient Registry: Relating and organising key details.
- Master language and reference data are described and structured in the data warehouse from a variety of source system details.
- The names, definitions and types of data are consistent with local requirements.
- The patient registries are determined solely by Implantable Cardioverter Defibrillator (ICD) billing information.
- The concept and implementation of patient registries and master data management are focused on data governance.

Level 3—Automated Internal Reporting

- Accurate, reliable performance automatic internal reporting: Automated internal reporting;
- The empirical motivation relies on the accurate and efficient production of reports promoting the basic operation and function of the healthcare organisation.
- Main performance indicators are conveniently available from the corporate level to the front-line boss.
- Data analysts from the corporate and company departments regularly collaborate to communicate and monitor.
- Data governance is expanding to enhance the organization's data literacy and to establish a data acquisition strategy for Level 4 and beyond.

Level 4—Automated External Reporting

- Efficient, reliable and agile development Automated external reporting:
- The empirical motivation relies on the accurate and efficient reporting required for regulatory and accreditation requirements.

- Compliance with industry-standard terms is required.
- Clinical text material is available for fast keyword searches.
- Unified data control operates for the review and approval of externally reported data.

Level 5—Waste and Care Variability Reduction

- Patient efficacy and accountable treatment evaluating and tracking evidence based care.
- The analytical purpose is to determine commitment to best clinical practice, minimize waste and reduce variability.
- Data governance is expanded to help care management teams focused on maximizing the health of the patient population.
- Population-based measurement is used to recommend individual health treatment upgrades.
- Permanent multidisciplinary teams are in position to continually manage prospects through emergency care procedures, chronic illnesses, patient protection situations and organizational workflows to maximize outcomes and reduce danger and cost.

Level 6—Population Health Management and Suggestive Analytics

- Population health management and recommended analytics: Take financial risk and educating community at the next level of study.
- The accountable organization of care shall bear the financial responsibility and reward associated with health outcomes.
- At least 50% of cases of emergency care shall be handled in the form of packaged payments.
- Analytics are available at the treatment point to help the triple target increase the quality of individual patient services, population control and the economy of care.
- Data content is expanded to include bedside controls, home monitoring data, external pharmacy data and costing depending on comprehensive service.
- Data regulation plays a critical role in maintaining the consistency of interventions that support doctors and executives with quality-based pay schemes.

Level 7—Clinical Risk Intervention and Predictive Analytics

- Taking more financial risk and proactively handling it.
- Medical risk intervention and statistical analysis.
- The methodological motivation is applied to fight diagnostic-based, fixed-fee per capita reimbursement models.
- Emphasis varies from case management to collaboration with physicians and payers to handle care episodes, leveraging statistical modelling, prediction, and risk stratification to promote outreach, triage, escalation, and referral.

- Doctors, clinics, employers, payers and members/patients collaborate together to share responsibility and reimburse (e.g., financial reward to patients for healthy behaviour).

Level 8—Personalized Medicine and Prescriptive Analytics

- Customized medication and prescriptive analytics contract with and regulating health.
- Analytical inspiration refers to health management, practical physical and emotional well-being, and mass customization of medication.
- Analytics is expanding to include email, prescriptive interpretation and guidance for intervention decisions.
- Prescriptive analyzes are required at the point of treatment to refine the clinical findings of patients on the basis of population data.
- Data content is expanded to cover data from 7 * 24 biometrics, genetic data and family data.

Level 9—Direct-to-Patient Analytics and AI Direct-to-patient analytics and AI

- Patients are expressly fitted with analytics and AI to ensure better personal ownership and precision of their health choices.
- Direct-to-patient analytics and AI are used in a collaborative decision-making process between patients and health professionals.
- Consumers, independent of insurance professionals, have the capacity to bring and analyze their whole health data ecosystem.
- The use of AI-based digital twins, "Patients like this" and "Patients like Me" pattern recognition is required for care and health management protocols.

4.3 Data Science Use Cases in Healthcare

Data-driven decision making opens up new options for the advancement of healthcare quality. A few handpicked cases of using data science in healthcare are described below.

Improve Diagnostic Accuracy

A variety of data analytics companies are now offering applications to providers by making use of sophisticated data analysis and machine learning methods to increase diagnostic accuracy [9]. Predictive analytics analyzes historical information, from patient records, health studies, signs, behaviours, diseases, genomic structure, etc., to accurately forecast the impact.

Make More Effective Use of EHR

A disruptive shift in the healthcare sector, and perhaps one of the widespread uses of big data, has been the availability of automated copies of patient records. EHR implementation has far-fetched advantages, such as reducing overheads, improving healthcare efficiency and streamlining processes [9]. The big data movement accelerating Innovation and Imagination' concerns a health-connected example that enables the exchange of data across all medical services and promotes the use of EHR.

Creation of Effective Pharmaceutical Drugs in a Shorter Period

It takes various procedures and several checks, and a lot of time and resources to discover a new prescription drug. Researchers will improve and shorten this method with the introduction of big data analytics. Data analytics and deep learning algorithms support study groups in any phase of the process by providing a data-driven viewpoint. It will forecast the success rate and how the compound will function in the human body, resulting in better drug development accuracy [9]. In order to learn how chemical molecules respond to alternative combinations of different cell types, genetic mutations, etc., quantitative drug exploration is often paired with genetic science. Data science applications are therefore a stimulus for biomedical discovery in a new age.

Reduce Risks in Prescription Medicine

Data science technology, aside from adding to diagnosis precision, also aims to reduce the risks inherent with pharmaceutical drugs [9]. Deep-learning algorithms equate it to the available databases and alert the doctor if it deviates from standard care procedures when a prescription is offered to the patient. By improving improved patient conditions and preventing deadly risks associated with expired prescriptions, this benefits the healthcare provider.

To Trigger Real-time Alerts

In-house healthcare is an expensive matter, as we have recognized, but tracking the patient's health statistics is much-needed for improved care. With the advent of wearable devices, doctors can virtually monitor the patient's vital statistics and, where applicable, offer real-time medical assistance [9]. Wearable devices collect and preserve care data in a cloud that is open to care management and practitioners. For example, the device warns the practitioner who may take immediate measures to save the patient anytime there is an alarming difference in a patient's blood pressure.

Improve Patient Engagement

A value-based treatment strategy is practiced by today's healthcare institutions, and patient participation plays a major role in it. Rising patient interest in the recovery plan has since become a top priority for healthcare providers. In order to fulfill the needs of the tech-savvy patient population, they spend mostly in designing techniques [9]. Healthcare professionals will easily bring big data analytics into motion to ensure that customers fully invest in their care. Artificial intelligence and interpretation of natural languages can be used to draw actionable conclusions and to create predictive risk scores to improve care collaboration. It deals mainly for patients who are subject to chronic illness treatment programs.

Streamline Knowledge Management

Problem-solving and achieving desired healthcare outcomes rely heavily on the knowledge bank. In the new healthcare environment, successfully balancing both existing expertise and externally gained knowledge is a concern for the provider [9]. A successful information management approach is important for delivering the best care available, ensuring organizational excellence and boosting creativity. It is easier to compile, archive, and spread different medical information through the introduction of big data into healthcare. Data science instruments are capable of combining data from various sources and analytics can be used by providers to produce optimum operating performance.

Simplify the Method of Internal Staffing

It is impossible for staffing management of any healthcare institution to decide the amount of workers needed at any given time. If the number of workers is higher than what is expected, it adds to the lack of labour, because if the employees are fewer, it leads to negative customer service ratings. It is possible to assess how many patients are at the hospital everyday and even hourly by taking advantage of statistical data [9]. Which aims to streamline the overall personnel management process, which contributes to shortened patient waiting times and increased quality of treatment?

Reduce Visits to Doctor

Mobile apps are also able to offer necessary healthcare assistance with the help of artificial intelligence. Instead of waiting for the doctor's visit, patients will explain symptoms, take tips and ask questions and recommendations from the insightful chat bots at any time. It offers regular updates about the medications and recovery plans and also helps to schedule a doctor's appointment [9]. For both patients and doctors, AI-based applications are advantageous. Although it saves doctors hours and can handle more urgent conditions, patients receive round-the-clock support. It encourages the patient to follow a healthier lifestyle that inevitably contributes to positive health outcomes.

Find a Treatment for Diseases

Many possible healthcare uses of data science are to identify drugs for dangerous diseases such as cancer, Ebola, etc. Researchers have an enormous array of evidence available on care programs, survival rates, illness effects, mortality, etc. They will uncover patterns and therapies that deliver high success rates in the real world with the use of data analytics technologies. Drug researchers, for example, can analyze the interaction between such mutations and cancer proteins and determine the best combination that will save the patient. In order to increase the quality of treatment, healthcare systems are constantly finding better options. It has introduced emerging innovations on a timely basis and aims to change towards a better future. Healthcare big data is a development in the making. The attitude of patients, doctors, and healthcare providers to treatment delivery has just begun to shift [2].

4.4 Data Analytics

Medical research has historically been a data-driven discipline, and with a gold standard in randomized clinical trials. However, medical science as well as clinical practice is increasingly evolving into Big Data-driven areas thanks to recent developments in medical imaging, integrated electronic health records and mobile devices. As such, the healthcare industry as a whole—physicians, customers, administrators, insurers and politics—will benefit greatly from the latest developments in Big Data technology and, in particular, analytics [9]. In order to develop specialized strategies and techniques for Big Data analytics in healthcare, there are many obstacles and needs. That contain as follows:

Multi-modal Data

There is an optimum collection of organized data in data processing, for example, as often seen in electronic health reports. However, a wide collection of unstructured information is a high percentage of health data. Many of them come in the form of real-time sensor readings, such as those for intensive care Electro Cardio Graph (ECG) scales, doctor's clinical note text data, and natural language medical literature, imaging data, or personalized medical data. It is necessary to obtain information from the data [4]. The goal should be to derive valuable knowledge from such heterogeneous data, to make it available to clinicians and to embed experience into the clinical records of patients.

Complex History Awareness

Quite specific phenomena need to be established by medical records; multi-level patient documentation on medical treatment and procedures, lifestyle information, a vast volume of medical evidence accessible in research, bio-banks, or research collections [10]. Therefore, in order to view data optimally, draw conclusions, identify acceptable interpretations and support clinical recommendations, medical data typically comes with complex metadata that needs to be taken into consideration.

Highly Skilled End-Users

Skilled end-users of medical diagnostic instruments, such as physicians, health practitioners and bioinformaticians are exceptionally available for different kind of analysis. They are also strongly responsible, meeting strong expectations of the consistency of diagnostic methods before putting their confidence in patient care. As far as possible, however, the optimal analytical approach should yield understandable patterns that allow for cross-checking findings and allow for trust in the solutions [6]. It can also allow expert self-service analytics and allow an expert to monitor the analytical process.

Privacy

Medical data is highly sensitive information that is secured by stringent legal safeguards at the European level. The availability of an appropriate regulatory system to allow the study of such data, as well as ample privacy-preserving computational tools to enforce this model, is critical for the functional usefulness and influence of data-driven medicine and health care [11].

Complex Decision Support

Imaging data analysis, intensive care surveillance, and pathology or multi-morbidity assessment is only a few reminders of how noisy data, dynamic situations, and potentially unreliable knowledge must be considered when making medical decisions. While neither humans nor algorithms are guaranteed to have the right solution, they may be forced to make crucial decisions or define alternatives in a limited period of time. Another area of medical decision-making assistance with possibly very high future consequences is smart supporters for patients who use smart phones, modern wearable technologies, and sensor networks to help patients track illness and lead a healthy life [12].

Any time-critical healthcare applications need to take steps right at a time where a dynamic event is detected in real-time analytics. Different sources of heterogeneous data have the ability to gain information in real time. There are several important, inter-connected approaches to this:

- Real-time analytics applies to analytics strategies that, when they enter a framework, can interpret and extract information from all obtainable data and tools in real time.
- Instead of storing and processing data for any point in the future, data stream mining refers to the ability to analyze and process streaming data at the moment.
- The detection and maintenance of patterns across multiple data sources relates to the dynamic recognition of situations where patterns are high-level, semantically rich, and essentially made visible to the user.

4.4.1 Future of Data Science in Healthcare

We believe that data mining will play a significant role in the growth of healthcare services. It is the primary capability that propels the development of precision medicine in the form of machine learning, and is generally regarded as a much-needed shift in healthcare. Although early attempts have proven difficult to provide diagnostic and care recommendations, we expect that data science will ultimately master that domain as well. For activities such as patient communication and recording of health information, speech and text recognition are still used and their use will increase. In all fields of health care, the greatest challenge for data science is not whether the technologies would be capable of being realistic enough, but rather to ensure that they are applied in routine clinical practice. Data science programs must be approved by authorities in order for uniform adoption, together with EHR schemes, to be standardized to a fair degree to ensure that similar products work equally, are taught to doctors, are paid by public or private paying entities and are updated on the market over time. At the end of the day, these hurdles will be overcome, but it will take far longer to do so than it will take to mature the systems themselves.

4.4.2 Stages of Analytics

Analytics is not a one-time effort or a sole attempt; it is an ongoing, evolving way of working that will adapt as the organization's expectations and priorities change. The more advanced phases of analytics provide skills that can assist with business planning, such as real-time insight and automated decision making, as well as forecasting. Predictive analytics examines historical data in order to forecast future target incidents. From a technology and business process standpoint, a company's journey into forward-looking analytics is a major transition.

Predictive analytics employs a variety of computational and machine learning techniques, which are refined over time as more evidence becomes available. The use of historical data from health reports together with external metrics such as weather forecasting and social media to calculate ER peak admissions in order to improve staff levels is an example of predictive analytics. Prescriptive analytics expands predictive analytics by including a basic or sequence of recommended behavior based on the prediction. The stages of analytics maturity are shown in Fig. 4.3.

Data methods such as modelling and deep learning as well as neural systems may be utilized by prescriptive solutions. Building upon the previous case, a prescriptive approach will develop a forecast for ER admissions peaks and then suggest changes to Workflow or prioritization to reduce the duration of stay and promise that as many patients as possible will be treated by workers. These guidelines may be focused on discrete business procedures or, in the case of cognitive systems, may be based on prior operations that have achieved an ideal outcome. Computer science tools such as artificial learning, deep learning and inference or logic systems are used for

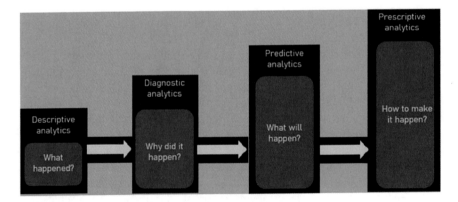

Fig. 4.3 Stages of analytics maturity

cognitive analytics. It uses human-like analysis to automate decisions or offer insights and recommendations to increase human choices. This will help to build a complete picture of the state of health of a patient, include everything from EMR reports to CT scans to the exercise tracker feed of the patient, and also provide the doctor with constructive, real-time advice on future medication choices or risk factors, and submit alerts to the patient with feedback on how to improve their well-being [4].

4.4.3   Healthcare Data Analytics Platforms

Different companies have deployed Artificial Intelligence (AI) programs to analyze textual data, written results, and image data to obtain significant outcomes in order to overcome healthcare big data problems and create smoother analytics. IBM Corporation is one of the biggest and most well-known providers of healthcare data analytics services. IBM's "Watson Health" is an AI portal that allows professionals, hospitals, and academics to share and interpret healthcare data [13]. Other major corporations, such as Oracle Corporation, Flatiron Health, and Google, are concentrating their efforts on developing distributed computational power systems for healthcare data analytics. Interestingly, in the recent few years, several companies and start-ups have also emerged to provide health care-based analytics and solutions. Some of the vendors in healthcare sector are provided in Table 4.1. Below we discuss a few of these commercial solutions.

4.4.4   Using Analytics to Address Chronic Disease Management

Many chronic diseases, such as diabetes, acute myocardial infarction, pneumonia and heart disease, have been classified as top priority by the Content Management System (CMS). They seek to slow down the rise in health care costs, in particular those related to patient referrals. Health history, cultural or socio-economic status and co-morbidities are some of the factors that affect the risk of having chronic disorders. Here is a short snapshot of each of these metrics [14]:

- Regular demographic records such as age, blood pressure, blood glucose levels, cholesterol levels and family history of clinical conditions are included in the patient's medical history. Statistical simulations use these data to assess disease progression and anticipate possible outcomes, helping doctors to decide about their treatment.
- The socio-economic and demographic factors play a crucial role in wellbeing. Variables such as ethnicity, income, educational level and even residential ZIP codes offer clues for the detection of patients at risk of chronic disease. This

Table 4.1 Companies which provide big data analysis services on healthcare domain [13]

Provider	Description
IBM Watson Health	For advanced research, it provides services for sharing clinical and health-related data among hospitals, academics, and providers
Mede analytics	Provides success improvement solutions, health programs and plans, and health monitoring, as well as patient results with a long track record
Health Fidelity	Provides a management solution for assessing risks in healthcare workflows, as well as optimization and modification approaches
Roam Analytics	Platforms for obtaining meaningful insights from large amounts of unstructured healthcare data
Flatiron Health	Applications are given for arranging and optimizing oncology data in order to enhance cancer care
Enlitic	Deep learning is provided for healthcare diagnosis using large-scale data sets from clinical studies
Digital Reasoning Systems	For analyzing and organizing unstructured data into usable data, the organization provides semantic computing services and data analytic solutions
Ayasdi	Platform with AI for therapeutic variations, population wellbeing, risk assessment, and other healthcare analytics
Linguamatics	Text mining tool for extracting valuable knowledge from unstructured healthcare data
Apixio	Provides a semantic processing tool for generating deep knowledge from clinical reports and pdf health records
Analytics of Roam	Provides infrastructure for natural language delivery in contemporary healthcare systems
Lumiata	Provides healthcare analytics and risk assessment systems to ensure effective results
Optum Health	Provides healthcare analytics, technology upgrades for modern health services, and robust and innovative healthcare technologies

expertise is not commonly available in a hospital, but can be accessed from a number of outlets, such as credit records, tax reports, and shopping patterns.

Finally, the medical hazard of patient is a feature of the various medical conditions a person may have. Hypertension and high cholesterol may be present in a patient being treated for diabetes and may be on several drugs to treat them both. These co-morbidities have an effect on decisions on care.

4.5 Prospective Analysis for Predictive Model

Effectively, prospective analysis tells us what is going to happen and gives you the chance to understand how you will be impacted in the future. In order to create associations and probable effects, it will take your data and then use a combination of algorithms and machine learning. This method of forecasting can help you better understand the needs of patients in healthcare, and gives you insight into admission trends, bed shortages, and several other challenges that can then be dealt with more effectively than ever from an administrative point of view. Prospective analytics helps assess what is extremely likely to happen in the future using prediction and forecasting techniques. These forecasts will then be used by doctors, researchers, medical specialty associations, pharmaceutical firms, and any other healthcare stakeholder to provide the best quality treatment for particular patients [9].

4.5.1 Future of Prospective Analysis for Predictive Model

Prospective analytics will become both more popular and more reliable as we amass more and more data. Currently, many quantitative models use standard statistical approaches that are useful and can produce informative outcomes, such as logistic regression. Data science and machine learning approaches such as random forests, however, can make more detailed forecasts when properly applied. Ultimately, Prospective analytics can take advantage of deep learning algorithms and can allow greater use of vast and diverse data sets as more feature-rich data is obtained and as the collection process itself progresses. A machine learning-based solution, on the other hand, would enable the radiologist to first extract all the features from the image. Deep learning simplifies the procedure by automatically identifying all the characteristics, without the radiologist doing additional effort. Simply put, big data and healthcare Prospective analytics go hand in hand, with more data indicating accurate forecasts. In order, to address its shortcomings, the field of Prospective analytics will progress. One current downside is that Prospective analytics cannot offer insight into what might happen following an operation or other transition, which can be problematic for researchers and clinicians who want to learn how patients could suffer after a new treatment or as a result of a new hospital procedure. We believe that Prospective analytics will progress beyond this challenge, enabling scientists to forecast the future in a far more detailed and holistic manner. The vast leaps in computer processing ability that make chewing through complex algorithms feasible would also be able to benefit from Prospective analytics.

4.5.2 Reliability in Analytics

Important decisions, often essentially life or death, must often be made in medical decision-making under the time constraints and in complicated and unclear circumstances with potentially harmful implications of mistakes if the correct decision is not taken. Although realizing that a data-driven approach cannot be 100% reliable, and also acknowledging that no doctor is inherently right, very high standards are needed for medical data analysis. Output assessment and monitoring (e.g. data-driven device accuracy) is also of paramount importance. This is not only a fundamental ethical principle, but unaddressed responsibility and safety concerns also impede the integration of new smart solutions into clinical practice. The key features of an empirical methodology that promotes trust in its practical implementation are comprehension in particular enabling individual physicians or researchers to be aware of its advantages and limitations; and reliability especially in the case of complex learning systems that evolve over time from a torrent of new input data, retaining reliability has been recognized as a major challenge [6].

4.5.3   Concerns of Prospective Analytics

Privacy

Ethical concerns regarding the use and misuse of data by businesses shouldn't come as much of a shock to decision makers. The increasing amount of data that is harvested by companies and the number of consumers who are cautious about it has meant that extra care must be taken by organizations handling large data sets. Many of these concerns have arisen from the sharp escalation of cyber attacks over the last few years, coupled with some disconcerting realities about preparedness.

Undermining Physicians

One of the enduring issues of the use of predictive analytics is the amount of deference that can be afforded to it and its role in the traditional decision making process that physicians undertake. For example, there may be significant legal ramifications if a doctor follows a predictive analytics model that is faulty or incorrect.

4.5.4   Benefits of Prospective Analysis

Advanced analysis methods are now focused on data to be observed, combined and analyzed from a number of sources. Many of these approaches provide statistical modelling capabilities that can provide clinicians with a range of inputs to address patient populations in an educated manner.

Operational Efficiency

When we talk about improving efficiencies within companies, Business Intelligence (BI) is also one of the greatest tools a company can have. BI is often used by them as a tool to move away from dubious gut-feeling decisions, and instead seeks to use current data for analytics and actionable data to make more educated decisions. Predictive analytics can be used to determine organizational inadequacies that may otherwise have been lost to a healthcare provider in terms of their importance.

Accuracy in Diagnosis and Preventative Care

Predictive analytics uses software to help physicians more accurately predict their patients in order to help resolve conditions before they arise. In order to provide a better understanding of the patient's journey, this is accomplished by analyzing data sets from hundreds, maybe thousands, of patients. This helps to provide an understanding of any problems they can have for diagnostic purposes, and then also allows physicians to better understand how well a patient responds to treatment. Using analytics in this way means that healthcare providers can intervene faster and facilitate patient trips more easily, more efficiently, and with an increased likelihood of a positive outcome.

4.6 Conclusion

In order to increase the quality of care, healthcare systems are constantly searching for better options. It has adopted emerging technology in a timely way and aims to develop for a better future. Data science and analytics has been used by the healthcare sector today to achieve comparative advantage by rising productivity and reducing costs. Data from healthcare is a revolution in the making. The way patients, doctors, and healthcare providers view the delivery of treatment has just begun to transform. Healthcare data and analytics are all set to become the revolutionary wave in the field of medical informatics with a vast amount of data produced each day. This chapter offers a comprehensive study to facilitating the accelerated growth, handling, analysis opportunities and challenges of healthcare data. There is also a need to monitor health care data, which is increasing at a fast pace from time to time and on a wider scale with lots of inconsistent data sources, in order to produce more effective outcomes from healthcare. Data science in healthcare data has the potential to revolutionize the healthcare industry by taking advantage of groundbreaking techniques of analytics.

References

1. J. Kaur, K.S. Mann, HealthCare platform for real time, predictive and prescriptive analytics using reactive programming. 10th Int. Conf. Comput. Electr. Eng. IOP Conf. Ser. J. Phys. Conf. Ser. **933**, 012010 (2018). https://doi.org/10.1088/1742-6596/933/1/012010
2. P. Nieminen, Applications of medical informatics and data analysis methods, MDPI. Appl. Sci. **10**, 7359 (2020)
3. D. Cirillo, A. Valencia, Big data analytics for personalized medicine. ScienceDirect Curr. Opin. Biotechnol. **58**, 161–167 (2019)
4. A. Bartley, Predictive Analytics in Healthcare, White Paper—Healthcare Predictive Analytics, ©Intel Corporation, Printed in USA 0917/FP/CAT/PDF 336536-001EN
5. D.W. Bates, S. Saria, L. Ohno-Machado, A. Shah, G. Escobar, Big data in health care: using analytics to identify and manage high-risk and high-cost patients. Health Aff. **33**(7), 1123–1131 (2014)

6. A. Kankanhalli, J. Hahn, S. Tan, G. Gao, Big data and analytics in healthcare: introduction to the special section. Inf. Syst. Front. **18**(2), 233–235 (2016)
7. S. Sinhasane, https://mobisoftinfotech.com/resources/blog/data-science-in-healthcare-use-cases (2019)
8. https://www.healthcatalyst.com/healthcare-analytics-adoption-model/
9. C. Birkmeye, *What is Predictive Analytics and Why is it Important? Healthcare Analytics* (ArborMetrix, 2020)
10. W. Raghupathi, V. Raghupathi, Big data analytics in healthcare: promise and potential. Heal. Inf. Sci. Syst. **2**(1), 3 (2014)
11. M. Ojha, K. Mathur, Proposed application of big data analytics in healthcare at Maharaja Yeshwantrao Hospital, in *3rd MEC International Conference on Big Data and Smart City (ICBDSC)*, 2016, pp. 1–7
12. G. Palem, *The Practice of Predictive Analytics in Healthcare*, https://www.researchgate.net/publication/236336250 (2013)
13. S. Dash, S.K. Shakyawar, M. Sharma, S. Kaushik, Big data in healthcare: management, analysis and future prospects. J. Big Data **6**(54) (2019)
14. A. Choudhury, B. Eksioglu, Using predictive analytics for cancer identification, in *Proceedings of the IISE Annual Conference*, eds. by H.E. Romeijn, A. Schaefer, R. Thomas (IISE, Orlando, 2019). Available at SSRN https://ssrn.com/abstract=3367567

Chapter 5
Emerging Advancement of Data Science in the Healthcare Informatics

Abstract The healthcare domain is experiencing a massive transition, driven by the threefold target of increased efficiency, reduced costs and positive results for patients. The lack of clinical experience impact can largely be due to inadequate statistical model effectiveness, difficulties understanding dynamic model forecasts, and lack of evidence from prospective clinical trials that have a strong benefit over the standard of treatment. In this article, the promise of personalized medicine's state-of-the-art data science methods, discussing open barriers, and Highlight paths that might in the future help to solve them. We should anticipate many shifts in future medical informatics science in view of the fluid existence of many of the driving factors behind advancement in knowledge management methods and their technology, developments in medicine and health care, and the constantly shifting demands, requirements and aspirations of human populations. This chapter gives brief explanation for relevance of the applications of predictive analytics strategies and importance of data science in healthcare.

Keywords Predictive analysis · Medical informative · Healthcare analysis · Data science

5.1 Introduction

Healthcare is perceived to be the main recipient of big data and analytics among many sectors. Data science has a significant role to play in the healthcare sector, from saving lives to cutting costs. The analysis of available evidence to assess which practices are most effective aims to reduce costs and improve the health of the people covered by health care providers by transferring health care to results and value-based payment programs [1]. As with the transition in time and improvements in technology, in order to increase the consistency, reliability and feasibility of patient services, there is a need to make systemic changes to health systems. It was expected that Electronic Health Reports and comprehensive data processing by health care providers would increase the efficacy and quality of patient care [2]. Statistics research refers

© The Author(s), under exclusive license to Springer Nature Singapore Pte Ltd. 2021   69
N. Thi Dieu Linh and Z. (Joan). Lu, *Data Science and Medical Informatics in Healthcare Technologies*, SpringerBriefs in Forensic and Medical Bioinformatics, https://doi.org/10.1007/978-981-16-3029-3_5

to the creation and implementation of instruments for planning, evaluating and inter-preting observational medical studies. The creative use of statistical inference theory, a clear understanding of clinical and epidemiological testing issues and an under-standing of the value of statistical software rely on the development of new statistical methods for medical applications [3]. Health care provides a wide variety of public and private data collection programs that provide multiple data bases. There are various applications of Data science in Healthcare showing in Fig. 5.1.

In almost every area, data analytics has become increasingly relevant. In the last century, the amount of evidence has grown exponentially as health care contributors switched to Electronic health Records (EHRs), digitized laboratory slides, videos and

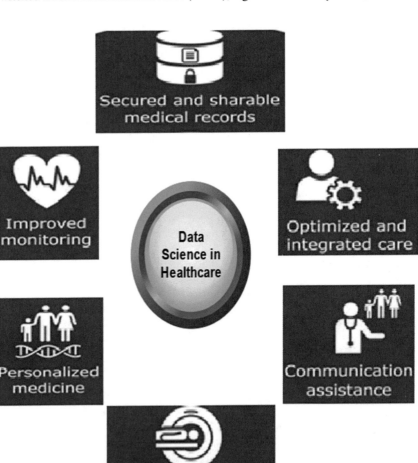

Fig. 5.1 Data science in healthcare

photographs of high-resolution radiology [4]. It is expected that data from genomics will expand substantially in the future as precision medicine is gradually incorporated into traditional clinical workflows. Patients create vast amounts of health data beyond the hospital atmosphere through the use of wearable fitness and exercise trackers and health applications. Huge data is also provided on a daily basis by the spread of health-related Internet of Things (IoT) devices, and also apps as well as other health-monitoring techniques. There is an immense ability for healthcare providers to combine these diverse sources and systems of data into new technologies. For example, additional resources such as social media or widely available government data need to be used to consider population health trends, in addition to the hospital's own archives. However, 94% of hospitals6 do not actually collect sufficient knowledge to perform effective public health analyzes [5].

5.1.1 What is Healthcare Analytics and Why Does It Matter?

If the estimated human lifespan expands, healthcare data collection of the world population is projected to make a major difference in modern medicine. Health analysis can theoretically reduce treatment costs, forecast epidemic outbreaks, circumvent preventable diseases, and ultimately improve the level of treatment and life of patients [6]. Big data essentially takes vast volumes of data, digitizes it and then consolidates it with a particular technology and analyzes it. In the case of health care analytics, the maxim "an ounce of prevention is worth a pound of cure" is incredibly accurate, since it will help doctors understand patients earlier in their lives, have early warning signs of disease, and manage illness in their early stages. Healthcare expenses accounted for 17.6% of GDP in 2018 after nearly 20 years of steady growth, nearly $600 billion higher than the estimated benchmark for a nation with the size and prosperity of the United States [7]. With prices beyond expectations, the healthcare sector wants data-driven solutions. Both healthcare providers and the economy benefit from these solutions. If more caregivers are paid on the basis of health results, there is a financial opportunity to reduce insurance providers' expenses while simultaneously enhancing patients' lives. And, given that medical decisions are most often made on facts, analysis and clinical data generated by healthcare analytics are in much higher demand [8].

5.1.2 Why Healthcare Analytics?

Data collection, data sharing, and data processing are three phases of data analysis that have slowed healthcare in the United States and other parts of the world. To date, the processing and delivery of data waves, which are marked by the urgent introduction of EHRs and medical information exchanges, have had little effect on healthcare efficiency and expense. In some cases, this nonstop data obsession has resulted in an over-focus on the EHR, resulting in contractor exhaustion and time and energy diverted from patients. Despite current hype about big data becoming the next "big" in other markets, we are only now getting the right predictive resources in healthcare to support quality assurance and cost-cutting measures around the sector. Healthcare analysis is the systematic use of data to generate useful information. The true promise of analytics lies in its ability to turn healthcare into some kind of data-driven environment powered by global analytics systems [7].

5.2 The Use of Data Science in Healthcare

Without a question, Machine Learning (ML), Computer Analysis, and Artificial Intelligence (AI) have been hot topics in all fields, including healthcare. Companies are racing to stock up on data scientists, big and small, but are data scientists alone adequate to create an effective healthcare data science practice, showing in Fig. 5.2. Data scientists are, without a doubt, essential to construct models. But you need a whole network of support functions to grow and maintain the team as you deal with healthcare and human data [9]. The large amounts of data which have been granted access to healthcare providers although the sector's digitalisation is referred to as big data in healthcare. Systematic review of these sets of data will yield actionable insights that will aid in making informed health-care choices. This seeks to establish a comprehensive and holistic viewpoint on patients, employers, and doctors.

Data science has the ability to locate all the data within a particular period and as needed. With regard to medicine, data science has tremendous importance because precision is a compulsory prerequisite of medicine. Data science helps healthcare industry stakeholders to provide a precise pool of data to operate on [11]. In both experimental innovation and clinical practice, there is always the potential to obtain

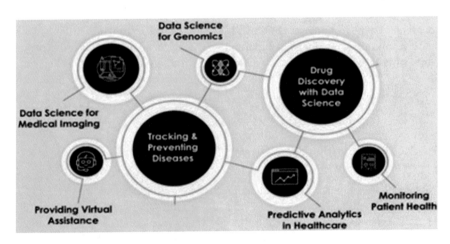

Fig. 5.2 Need for data science in healthcare [10]

precise curate data that is of great value. At the correct time and place, it is always possible to keep an eye on the latest developments in the health of the patient through data science interventions. A reliable and consistent flow of information must always be maintained such that the organization's equilibrium is maintained and care can be completed effectively. In healthcare, there are many data science applications [10].

Use of Data Science in Preventive Imaging

The pre-treatment diagnostic process is one of the main stages of the use of data science in healthcare. In the field of medicine, cutting edge precision is of utmost importance because the entire treatment protocol and the patient's recovery are highly dependent on the accuracy of the initial physiological and symptomic data gathered. Data science is strongly related to AI. In reality, AI is the central force behind the collection of specific data for patients. This precision also allows physicians to prescribe personalized preventive medication according to the patient's needs. This is particularly helpful in situations where the patient is pregnant or has a raging tumour. Therapy based on non-intrusive medicine is of utmost importance in such a situation. This makes patient efforts pro-active and contributes greatly to making the experience of treatment both satisfactory and soothing.

Use of Data Science in Genomics

A relatively new field of medical science is MODERN Genomics. In order to do away with fatal or painfully intolerable genetic disorders, the study of genes focuses on estimating the need for medical intervention. There is a sure shot solution for all of these with the rise of medical science and therefore it is possible to take timely measures to save a lot of precious lives with the aid of data science in genomics. Genetic activity data is typically unpredictable and produces a situation of uncertainty in flux. AI allows genomic specialists to take concrete steps to help improve patient wellbeing.

Virtual Assistance with Data Science

In order to provide virtual assistance to patients in need, data science is of great importance. This is of particular significance in situations where an immediate emergency arises. There are cases of pre-mature delivery or erratic and untimely seizures that need urgent intervention to save the victim's life. The same is the case with individuals who have been trapped in a fire or witnessed a traumatic incident such as rape, theft or break-in with some other malicious intent. There are also a number of areas where having medical infrastructure is very difficult and yet these places are populated. It is in such a situation that virtual support is of high importance. Most significantly, it saves the lives of individuals who are lucky enough to be protected by virtual medical care.

Predictive Analytics in Healthcare

There is ample medical evidence to establish that individuals in a certain age group are affected by particular varieties of diseases. This is not to suggest that the patterns are uniformly the same, but that there are some indicators that help doctors discover a specific group's tendency to fall victim to a particular disease. Data analyses of past cases and patient identification of current patients will help doctors raise awareness among the general population and inculcate behaviours that are more health-friendly for people.

Data Science in Neuro Care

In the field of neurocare, data science has a major role to play. It is no secret that in its conclusions, data science is precise and its outcomes are more than just credible in the hands of quality data analysts. In order to bring about efficient and effective neuro treatment, they help to create insights into the potential course of action. The brain is an intricate organ and perhaps the most important aspect of a human being's life. For individuals suffering from these conditions, minute sensory or motor nerve symptoms may be life-threatening. Thus, AI is very important as a method for improving patients' neurological wellbeing and offering a sense of certainty to the ailing. If physicians have specific data with them as an outcome of proactive data science initiatives, major brain operations can be conducted efficiently.

Data Science and Effective Dieting

We live in an era in which patterns of consumption have become a raging issue. Therefore, it is very critical that the new advances in data science add value to dieting efforts. Data obtained from various sources regarding people's lifestyle habits can be beneficial by splitting them into different categories to establish unique diet routines for different types of people. According to the analyzed data, it is also possible for doctors to recommend accurate diets, whether it is an actual patient history or a record of people who have suffered a similar problem in the past.

Data Science and Psychology

Psychology is an area of medical science that focuses very much on the unique case data of an individual patient, despite its apparent universality. It is here that AI within permissible period assists in quality psychoanalysis and psychoanalytic treatment.

The Healthcare Analytics Adoption Model

Without a vision and goal-driven framework [7], health data and analytics can be intimidating and overwhelming. The healthcare analytics adoption model was created by a consortium of cross-industry healthcare veterans because the healthcare industry lacked a comprehensive analytics model that addressed the unique demands of health data [7]. Throughout their analytical journey, health institutions should turn to the model as it offers comprehensive guidelines on the classification of analytical capability classes and provides standardized sequencing within the health system for the application of analytics. Some type of an analytical model is critical for health systems because the right model will lay the foundations for a feasible, competitive analytics solution that will address more complex data needs in the future..

5.3 Emerging Approaches to Advance Healthcare Data Analytics

While multiple studies have reported the opportunity for Data Analytics in healthcare, the future risks resulting from the use of such instruments have received equal attention. Data processing in the field of medicine and chronic disease management, to population wellbeing and precision medicine has proven its potential in growing various health care fields [12]. These algorithms could boost the quality of health care, reduce logistical burdens and speed up the diagnosis of diseases. Although these methods can be healthy, the harm caused by such algorithms is just as high. The use of these resources in daily healthcare is hampered by questions over data access and processing, unconscious and overt bias as well as difficulties with the patient and provider faith. Health experts and service organizations collaborate towards identifying solutions to these challenges, while promoting the use of data analytics for greater outcomes and results of health treatment [13].

Providing Comprehensive, Quality Training Data

In healthcare, the effectiveness of data analytics tools is generally understood to rely on the value of the knowledge used to train them. Inaccurate, low quality data-trained algorithms can produce incorrect results, leading to insufficient treatment.

However, it is difficult, time-consuming to acquire quality training data which enables multiple companies to develop successful models without the resources needed. Healthcare officials have also been inspired by the ongoing healthcare crises to develop quality, clean datasets for algorithm development. The dataset can be used to enhance machine learning algorithm preparation, allowing anatomical structures to be identified in new scans.

Reducing Bias in Data and Algorithms

When healthcare providers are increasingly dependent on computational algorithms to assist them in making treatment decisions, it is important that these technologies are free of unconscious or overt bias that could push health inequities further. Given the current differences that pervade the healthcare sector, it is also impossible to create perfect, bias-free algorithms. Although it is incredibly important to connect with providers and end-users during algorithm development, this stage is sometimes only half the fight. It's a time-consuming, challenging challenge to gather the high-quality data needed to build unbiased analytics tools.

Developing Quality Tools While Preserving Data Privacy

The topic of data protection and protection is high on the list of issues in algorithm development. Researchers may avoid accessing the broad, varied data sets required to train analytics technology across legal, privacy, and cultural barriers. Traditional machine learning approaches include a centralized database where patient data can be obtained directly for a machine learning model's preparation. Practical challenges such as patient safety, identity management, data ownership, and the pressure on hospitals that must build and manage these consolidated databases influence such approaches. Clinicians may train an algorithm through several clustered devices or repositories containing local data samples without sharing them, using an evolving technique called federated learning.

Ensuring Providers Trust and Support Analytics Tools

It is important for patients to trust that analytics algorithms can keep their data secure, it is essential for clinicians to trust that knowledge can be delivered in a valuable, trustworthy manner through these tools. Additionally, leaders could utilize AI instruments at the point of treatment to improve clinical decision-making. Allowing patients to study and develop AI tools will also help ensure that the technology is onboard for clinicians. With healthcare organisations rapidly leveraging data analytics technologies for better insights and simplified treatment processes, it will be vital for the effective use of these models in clinical care to address problems of bias, privacy and protection, and consumer confidence.

5.3.1 Data Analytics in Healthcare

It would be easier to compile medical information through data analytics in healthcare and convert it into concrete and usable insights that can then be used to offer improved services. Here are a few examples of how healthcare analytics can be used to predict and prevent challenges before they are too late, as well as to evaluate current procedures, effectively include patients with their own healthcare, pace up and maximize medication, and track inventory more specifically. Seven Ways in which data analytics changes the healthcare industry [14].

Heath Tracking

Among the most significant advancements in healthcare are big technology, science, and the Internet of Things (IoT). Wearable sensors, which are mounted to our bodies, will help to monitor the condition of our bodies in the future. This gives doctors a better understanding of how the body works over time. This also suggests that hospitalization, which saves money, is not needed for monitoring.

Reducing Costs

Failure to determine how many staff needs to be in the hospital leads to either over or understaffing. We can be more consistent with our assessment by means of analytics. We may also enhance the distribution of personnel. We can then determine the personnel required for each organization precisely. In addition, we will approximate the number of beds needed to accommodate patients. This will prevent hospitalization from keeping patients on waiting lists.

Assisting High-risk Patients

Analytics are ideal for determining the needs of high-risk and chronic patients. In the context of corrective steps to minimize the need for repeated hospital visits, this will help doctors come up with improved treatment approaches.

Preventing Human Errors

Doctors treat huge numbers of patients on a regular basis in certain cases. This may contribute to fatigue, which in turn contributes to errors. Big data and its monitoring software can help flag possible errors and prevent potentially catastrophic errors.

Advancement in Healthcare Sector

We can also use large data analysis to sift through vast databases in order to find solutions to complicated medical issues. The more testing we do, the larger these libraries get, and doctors will be able to solve complex medical problems in moments. In less time than ever before, healthcare research can become more structured and relevant.

Wearable Device Data to Prevent and Monitor Healthcare Problems

Each day, human body produces approximately 2 terabytes of information. We can record much of it with current wearable technology. The race for medical monitoring by wearable has been joined by several big technologies and technology brands. The ability for such analytics to be implemented is impressive. Strokes, Heart attacks and other possibly fatal health conditions should be predicted and responded to in real time. This implies that we'll be able to save lives in addition to getting a diagnosis. Wearable technology will also help people change their diets in order to prevent potential and ongoing health issues.

Improving Diagnostic Accuracy and Efficiency

Patients misdiagnosed are not a phenomenon of the past. Enlitic is a start-up that seeks to enhance diagnosis accuracy by in-depth learning. This is made possible by an algorithm that is capable of manipulating image images. This includes CT scans, x-rays and other imaging data. This technology can also be used to avoid the misdiagnosis of serious illnesses that are normally ignored.

5.3.2 Outlook of Data Science in Healthcare Domain

We believe that data mining will play a significant role in the growth of healthcare services. It is the empowerment approach that propels precision medicine forward in the context of machine learning, which is generally acknowledged as a key treatment transition [7]. Although early attempts have proven difficult to provide diagnostic and care recommendations, we expect that data science will ultimately master that domain as well. It seems likely that much of the X-ray and pathological images will be processed by a computer at some point, taking into account rapid advances in data technology for image processing. For activities such as patient communication and recording of health information, speech and text recognition are still used and their use will increase. In all fields of health care, the greatest challenge for data science is not whether the technologies would be capable of being realistic enough, but rather to ensure that they are applied in routine clinical practice. Data science programs must be approved by authorities in order for uniform adoption, together with EHR schemes, to be standardized to a fair degree to ensure that similar products work equally, are taught to doctors, are paid by public or private paying entities and are updated on the market over time. At the end of the day, these hurdles will be overcome, but it will take far longer to do so than it will take to mature the systems themselves.

5.4 Importance of Advanced Analytics in Healthcare

One of the most important advances in health care as a whole in recent years has been the application of Data mining for health insurance. The first shift can be seen in the expanded usability of both organized and unstructured content. We now have unprecedented access to knowledge thanks to cloud computing, artificial intelligence, and analytics [16]. Better decision-making, reduced costs, and increased accessibility are all benefits of using this technology in healthcare. The healthcare organization's leadership recognised the importance of these scientific advances. There are three main ways for health care organisations to use this method of data processing:

1. Improved development of pipeline R&D
2. Improvement of methods for diagnosis and rehabilitation
3. Better implementation of detection and monitoring

There are some fundamental analytical layers important to the healthcare sector [15]:

- Promotion of commerce
- Asset analytics for medical devices
- Operation review for medical equipment
- Analytics for social media
- Management of clinical data Compliance to invest

All will be confused by the vast amount of data that appears to flow across healthcare networks every second of the day. However, learning practical lessons from it and using them to treat patients and prevent illness is a huge step forward in healthcare. The data you get on your computers is a jumble of zeros and ones, and you can't do something about it until you figure out what you're supposed to say. According to the wellbeing trigger report, 90% of respondents accepted that analytics would be "highly relevant" or "very important" to their organization in the coming years. Respondents weighed in on the importance of health advances, as well as the part analytics plays in them. Analytics is becoming increasingly relevant for tracking various facets of health-care developments. Advanced scientific discipline concerned with the area of including clinical, corporate, health information technology and financial areas.

5.4.1 The Value of Data in Analytics

The practice of analyzing all the data collected from different sources is known as healthcare data management. This helps healthcare providers to treat their patients holistically, deliver personalized services, and improve health outcomes. The health-care industry has become more dynamic and complex, and it is becoming more difficult. Efficient tools and methods are needed to extract value from data. The available technologies will assist you in making informed decisions by collecting data and leading to increased healthcare outcomes. Organizations are given a lot of details to help them find out what the patient's needs are. When they review the analytics, they gain a better understanding of the patient's diagnosis, allowing them to deliver precision-driven care and treatment. This invariably leads to end-to-end process management and increased efficiency.

5.4.2 Analytics for Transforming Healthcare

Throughout the United States, healthcare organizations have been implementing technologies such as Picture Archiving And Communication System (PACS) imaging systems, tele-health systems, and EMRs (electronic medical records) to try to make sense of the massive amount of data flowing through the system (both structured and unstructured). As a result, learning what approaches are capable of obtaining knowledge from the findings is important in order to generate value and enjoy organizational, economical, and clinical perspectives. Genome analyzers and other research methods assist in the understanding of consumer evidence and the retrieval of unwanted/unnecessary information in order to achieve what is desired. The patient will benefit from improved fitness as a result of this. Data gathered from multiple databases can be used in a number of ways by healthcare organisations.

Disease Surveillance and Preventative Management

To detect any patterns, both structured and unstructured data is scanned, including material readily available on non-traditional sites such as social media updates, text messages, and the like. All of the evidence were translated into actionable insights that are used to enhance patient conditions. In this respect, the proliferation of smart devices has made a significant difference. It helps researchers to predict the distribution of communicable diseases (through the GPS coordinates obtained from the cell phone). This is how they were able to take precautions during the West African Ebola epidemic. Data on smartphone travel will give insight on diseases that could spread in the future, in addition to making us understand recent cases of pathogens and infectious diseases. The data use and conversion process [16]:

- To examine the trends in the data and keep an eye out for epidemic outbreaks. Caregivers must be able to provide medication as well as conduct a thorough examination in the event of a medical emergency.
- Improving prevention approaches, medications, and vaccines by analyzing the data.
- Study to avoid the epidemic from spreading and to mitigate disease-related fatalities by testing where emergency treatment is required.

Develop More Effective Diagnostic and Therapeutic Techniques

Organizations rely on the experience of healthcare analytics to collaborate to monitor the success of their processes through data obtained from different sources. This will help them understand how their initiative has been reacted to by the patients and what their situation is now. Here are several fields where predictive analytics and healthcare informatics will support healthcare providers:

- Recognizing people that are at risk of developing diseases or other health problems.
- Develop personalized wellbeing programs to meet the needs of patients in order to improve their fitness.
- Recognize redundant processes and methods that do not produce the desired results and discard them entirely. This means that the health program kits only contain results-oriented services. The majority has been omitted.
- The patient may need to be readmitted in certain circumstances due to a relapse or an adverse effect. The analytics will be able to identify the cause of the relapse and make predictions on how to prevent it.
- After study, it is possible to maximize resource use, increase efficiency, and increase throughput.

Although predicting health outcomes using both peer-reviewed journals and sources, the analytics would also take into account the most recent medical research. The forecasts will be accompanied by analysis that the human brain will never be able to perceive or presume. This is why predictions differ depending on how the patient reacts to hospital referrals for drugs [16]. The success profile acquired from previous patients is also developed using artificial intelligence. This technique is used to build a prediction model. After that, this procedure is used to assist prospective patients in receiving a new diagnosis.

Development of a More Productive and Faster R&D Pipeline

Getting the medication out to the patient is not easy. In order to produce the drug, there is a lengthy and overwhelming process, bringing it through elaborate clinical trials and then, eventually, Food and Drug Administration (FDA) approval. Prior to prescribing medications to patients, any pharmaceutical organization and healthcare service provider must go through this practice. To shorten the time a drug spends in the R&D pipeline, businesses use predictive modelling, computational methods and algorithms, and healthcare analytics. Below, the benefits are stated:

- In building a quick leaner and highly efficient R&D pipeline, advanced analytics play an important role.
- Searching for methods to accelerate the drug discovery process in order to improve patient wellbeing. Try procedures that avoid errors in clinical trials and strengthen the processes of patient recruitment.
- Review patient records to see if medication reactions have happened in the past, as new medications have been placed on the market, and to determine the effects of these drugs.

In order to have a very fast and effective pipeline, healthcare institutions need to have advanced software and strategies to better analyze all the knowledge that comes in.

5.4.3 The Significance of Analytics in Various Fields

The healthcare sector is undergoing extreme metamorphic changes as it transforms from a volume-based business to a value-added company. Value-based medicine puts a lot of emphasis on healthcare providers to have better outcomes for patients. As a result, cost systems have improved, life expectancy has increased, and chronic illnesses and infectious diseases have become better controlled. Many other organisations have been impacted by the benefits, including healthcare companies, insurance providers, government agencies, and so on. Insurance providers, for example, use fee-for-service models to transition to value-based, data-driven payments. Electronic medical records may offer high-quality patient care. Together, all these bodies are associated with these areas:

Disease Prevention and Intervention

Analytics is also used in disease control and prevention approaches. Organizations would be able to recognise patients at high risk of developing chronic illnesses early on and have better treatment so that they do not have to deal with long-term health issues. Avoid the need for long-term therapy, which could require the use of long-acting medications and potential side effects.

Care Coordination

Analytics helps to provide continuity of treatment and this is really useful in intensive care. Particularly when rapid response time is required. This can save the life of the patient. In a 30-day timeframe, analytics can also warn the caretaker to deploying care management strategies.

Customer Service

In healthcare, excellent service is extremely critical, and any inconsistencies in service could produce serious problems. Customer service can be profoundly influenced by analytics. And it lets you have a personalized touch, correctly perceive the needs of the patient and also motivates them to enhance their wellness. The customized approach given by analytics can really help the clinician achieve better results.

Financial Risk Management

Artificial Intelligence is the key to liquidity risk management. As per the clinicians & healthcare networks report, the biggest financial obstacle to the fee-for-service success contract paradigm is that determining patient conditions and settling on payment takes a long time. Such roadblocks include lower reimbursements, deferred patient bills, underutilized billing, and underutilized record monitoring technology. Predictive modeling will aid cash flow to hospitals by assessing which accounts need to be charged and forecasting which bills are likely to stay unpaid in the hospital.

Fraud and Abuse

In detecting fraud and violence, using data and analytics will help. There may be many examples of fraudulent healthcare accidents, ranging from honest errors such as incorrect billings, wasteful medical tests, false statements that lead to illegal payments, and so on. Healthcare big data helps to recognise the trends leading to possible fraud patterns and even to comply with health insurance. Sniffing out false statements is not the boring phase it once was anymore.

Operations

Healthcare has gradually begun to focus on technologies to guide the decision-making process. With advanced technological technology and adequate data processing, they would be able to make important operational decisions. They also began to move away from a reactive approach to patient traffic control, encouraging the removal of systemic bottlenecks and the reduction of clinical differences. As a result of being able to draw straightforward information from evidence from the health sector, organizations have managed to make sound decisions.

Healthcare Reform

Health organizations are in a position to drive health-care changes by analytics, and this would, in essence, contribute to an unprecedented amount of restructuring reimbursement. This is powerful enough to bring in drastic improvements by making it deliver, not quantity, but importance, and not service, but efficiency, in the current hospital delivery model.

5.5 Data Analytics Using Predictive Model in Healthcare

The use of predictive analytics model for healthcare organization is one of the biggest transformative developments in medicine today [17]. In particular, this suggests the use of healthcare data in much the same way as it is used by banks to predict the types of loans that are ideally suited to specific clients. Yet healthcare data can be used in medicine to assess. In this way, data analytics will enhance patient treatment, patient satisfaction and costs. It will scan for vast quantities of data not available to medical professionals at their fingertips. And, even though they do, in order to make better choices, they do not have time to evaluate and incorporate the conditions of particular patients.

5.5.1 Benefits of Predictive Model in Healthcare [18]

Improved Preventive Medicine and Public Health

Now it is known, how significant early intervention, especially in the field of genomics, is in preventing or reducing disease severity. When patients and their physicians realize the risks, it is possible to make behavioural adjustments through healthcare informatics, and treatment/monitoring protocols may begin sooner. In exchange, this would save medical costs. In fact, the entire area of genomics is a perfect location for health predictive analytics to use cases for preventive purposes.

Cuts-down Healthcare Costs

As an additional benefit, many organizations provide their workforce with healthcare. Using the predictive algorithm, they can input the characteristics and data of their workers and get estimates of potential costs. They will also work with insurance firms who already have their own statistical data algorithms. Predictive analytics can be used by employers to make decisions about which insurance provider can better suit their needs. In order to integrate databases and then use predictive analysis to create better insurance products for a specific workforce, a company and hospitals can cooperate with insurance companies. This is where predictive empirical usage cases in healthcare will help all.

The Ultimate Beneficiaries—Patients

Using predictive analytics will potentially improve the treatment of patients. People will receive protocols of care that specifically function with them. They will use precisely targeted drugs based on their particular characteristics and will be made aware of health hazards sooner so that preventive therapies and improvements in lifestyle can occur. Patients would, in short, be more educated. And recent surveys have shown that patients, including senior citizens, are open to being part of the technologies and data collecting needed to achieve safer, individualized and more cost-effective healthcare.

5.5.2 Clinical Predictive Analytics Market

Using predictive analytics will potentially improve the treatment of patients. People will receive protocols of care that specifically function with them. They will use precisely targeted drugs based on their particular characteristics and will be made aware of health hazards sooner so that preventive therapies and improvements in lifestyle can occur. Patients would, in short, be more educated. And recent surveys have shown that patients, including senior citizens, are open to being part of the technologies and data collecting needed to achieve safer, individualized and more cost-effective healthcare.

- Has valuable expertise in software applications for healthcare.
- Provides solid layers of visualization for readability.
- Set up impenetrable detection systems.
- Provides a superior ETL method (extract, transform, and load) to download and location data from databases in others.
- Provides you only what you need at the moment, but provides ongoing assistance and expansion as these needs arise.

5.5.3 Concerns of Predictive Analytics

Privacy

Ethical concerns regarding the use and misuse of data by businesses shouldn't come as much of a shock to decision makers. The increasing amount of data that is harvested by companies and the number of consumers who are cautious about it has meant that extra care must be taken by organizations handling large data sets. Many of these concerns have arisen from the sharp escalation of cyber attacks over the last few years, coupled with some disconcerting realities about preparedness.

Undermining Physicians

One of the enduring issues of the use of predictive analytics (or any AI tech for that matter) is the amount of deference that can be afforded to it and its role in the traditional decision making process that physicians undertake. For example, there may be significant legal ramifications if a doctor follows a predictive analytics model that is faulty or incorrect.

5.5.4 Benefits of Predictive Analytics

Advanced analytics tools are now based on data to be observed, combined and analyzed from a variety of sources. Many of these methods have predictive modelling capabilities that can provide physicians with a variety of inputs to target patient groups in an informed manner.

Operational Efficiency

When we talk about improving efficiencies within companies, business intelligence is also one of the greatest tools a company can have. BI is often used by them as a tool to move away from dubious gut-feeling decisions, and instead seeks to use current data for analytics and actionable data to make more educated decisions. Predictive analytics can be used to determine organizational inadequacies that may otherwise have been lost to a healthcare provider in terms of their importance.

Accuracy in Diagnosis and Preventative Care

In order to better address problems before they occur, predictive analytics uses tools to help doctors anticipate their patients more accurately. This is done by reviewing data sets from hundreds, maybe thousands, of patients in order to provide a clearer understanding of the patient's journey. This helps to provide an overview of any diagnostic concerns they may have, which then allows doctors to better understand how well a patient responds to care. Using analytics in this way ensures that healthcare providers can intervene more effectively, more reliably, and with an increased probability of a positive result more quickly and encourage patient trips. In this case, it must be stressed that no algorithm is supposed to replace a physician. Rather, the idea should be to provide them with a mechanism at hand that can help their decisions on the basis of rational, data-driven criteria and the abundance of biomedical information available.

5.6   Conclusion

This chapter offers a systematic overview of precision healthcare that affects the gains of data analytics and techniques of quantitative analysis. It offers a comprehensive approach to facilitating the accelerated growth, handling and study of medical evidence. This has also been demonstrated that the healthcare industry has certain very unique features, prospects, and threats that necessitate concentrated attention and study to fully realize their potential. In order to deliver more reliable healthcare services, there is also a need to track health care data, which is growing at a rapid rate from time to time and on a larger scale with many unreliable data outlets. This will be accomplished by placing data analysis technology at the centre of their efforts, with the goal of seeing their findings scaled up and embraced by the entire healthcare industry.

References

1. M. Ojha, K. Mathur, Proposed application of big data analytics in healthcare at Maharaja Yeshwantrao Hospital, in *3rd MEC International Conference on Big Data and Smart City (ICBDSC)*, 2016, pp. 1–7
2. J. Kaur, K.S. Mann, HealthCare platform for real time, predictive and prescriptive analytics using reactive programming. 10th Int. Conf. Comput. Electr. Eng. IOP Conf. Ser. J. Phys. Conf. Ser. **933**, 012010 (2018). https://doi.org/10.1088/1742-6596/933/1/012010
3. P. Nieminen, Applications of medical informatics and data analysis methods, MDPI. Appl. Sci. **10**, 7359 (2020)
4. A. Kankanhalli, J. Hahn, S. Tan, G. Gao, Big data and analytics in healthcare: introduction to the special section. Inf. Syst. Front. **18**(2), 233–235 (2016)
5. A. Bartley, Predictive Analytics In Healthcare, White Paper—Healthcare Predictive Analytics, ©Intel Corporation, Printed in USA 0917/FP/CAT/PDF 336536-001EN
6. W. Raghupathi, V. Raghupathi, Big data analytics in healthcare: promise and potential. Heal. Inf. Sci. Syst. **2**(1), 3 (2014)
7. https://www.healthcatalyst.com/healthcare-analytics-adoption-model/
8. R. Chauhan, R. Jangade (2016) A robust model for big healthcare data analytics, in *6th International Conference—Cloud System and Big Data Engineering (Confluence)*, pp. 221–225
9. S. Sinhasane, https://mobisoftinfotech.com/resources/blog/data-science-in-healthcare-use-cases (2019)
10. http://www.primeclasses.in/blog/2019/08/26/the-need-for-data-science-in-healthcare-industry/
11. D.W. Bates, S. Saria, L. Ohno-Machado, A. Shah, G. Escobar, Big data in health care: using analytics to identify and manage high-risk and high-cost patients. Health Aff. **33**(7), 1123–1131 (2014)
12. H. Asri, H. Mousannif, H. Al Moatassime, T. Noel, Big data in healthcare: challenges and opportunities. Proc. Int. Conf. Cloud Comput. Technol. Appl. CloudTech. (2015)
13. BDV, TF7 Healthcare Subgroup, *Big Data Technologies in Healthcare: Needs, Opportunities and Challenges* (2016)
14. http://starbridgepartners.com/2019/10/why-is-data-analytics-important-in-healthcare/
15. https://www.cabotsolutions.com/importance-of-advanced-analytics-in-healthcare
16. R. Ding, M.L. McCarthy, J. Lee, J.S. Desmond, S.L. Zeger, D. Aronsky, Predicting emergency department length of stay using quantile regression. Int. Conf. Manage. Serv. Sci. **45**(2), 1–4
17. C. Birkmeye, *What is Predictive Analytics and Why is it Important? Healthcare Analytics* (ArborMetrix, 2020)
18. A. Choudhury, B. Eksioglu, Using predictive analytics for cancer identification, in *Proceedings of the IISE Annual Conference*, eds. by H.E. Romeijn, A. Schaefer, R. Thomas (IISE, Orlando, 2020). Available at SSRN https://ssrn.com/abstract=3367567

Printed in the United States
by Baker & Taylor Publisher Services